Music in Therapeutic Practice

Music in Therapeutic Practice

Using Rhythm to Bridge Communication Barriers

Trisha Ready

ROWMAN & LITTLEFIELD
Lanham • Boulder • New York • London

Published by Rowman & Littlefield
A wholly owned subsidiary of The Rowman & Littlefield Publishing Group, Inc.
4501 Forbes Boulevard, Suite 200, Lanham, Maryland 20706
www.rowman.com

Unit A, Whitacre Mews, 26-34 Stannary Street, London SE11 4AB

Copyright © 2016 by Rowman & Littlefield

All rights reserved. No part of this book may be reproduced in any form or by any electronic or mechanical means, including information storage and retrieval systems, without written permission from the publisher, except by a reviewer who may quote passages in a review.

British Library Cataloguing in Publication Information Available

Library of Congress Cataloging-in-Publication Data Available

ISBN: 978-1-4422-3620-2 (cloth : alk. paper)
ISBN: 978-1-4422-3621-9 (electronic)

∞™ The paper used in this publication meets the minimum requirements of American National Standard for Information Sciences—Permanence of Paper for Printed Library Materials, ANSI/NISO Z39.48-1992.

Printed in the United States of America

Contents

Acknowledgments		vii
1	Introduction	1
2	Metaphors of Music: A Literature Review	7
3	Music and Bonding	17
4	Blue Eyes, Bread, and Water	25
5	Imaginary Nightclub as Potential Space	37
6	Ramble On: Raves, Social Urges, and Psychosis	49
7	Wrote on Your Wall Before Leaving	63
8	Play Marshall Mathers, Please	73
9	Conclusion	83
Bibliography		89
Index		109
About the Author		117

Acknowledgments

I am grateful to the individuals who have allowed me to understand their intimate relationships to music, particularly the participants in the music listening sessions, without whom I would not have begun this inquiry in earnest. (Their identities have been altered to honor their privacy.) I hope the question of how to use patient self-selected music to promote shared, humane exploration and engagement continues on as an active inquiry for readers.

A sincere thanks to Allen Bishop of Pacifica Graduate Institute and the Reiss Davis Child Study Center for his generous guidance, support, and inspiration, and to Dr. James Grotstein and Christine Lewis for their reflections and reveries.

Thanks to Dr. William Adams, O'Donnell Day, Amy Cummings Garcia, Shahzina Karam, and Gerri Pergola for their initial encouragement in the integration of music into hospital programming. Thanks to the dedicated staff at Fairfax Hospital, including Ron Escarda, John Beall, Richard Geiger, Ann Schreiber, Annalisa Shark, Jen Drake, and Todd Thoma, as well as Debbie Horowski.

Thanks to the judges of the Division 39 Johanna K. Tabin Book Prize for honoring an early draft of chapter 4, and particularly to Henry M. Seiden for encouraging me to pursue publication. My deepest gratitude goes out to Dr. Seiden as well as Marilyn Charles, Michael O'Loughlin, Sandra Ullman, Selena Gray, Terri Stuart, and Joan Lam for their ongoing confidence and kindness.

Profound thanks to Frith Maier for enduring the writing process, and for her fine mind for details—cracks in climbing rocks, crevasses, and commas. Tina Kelley and Cristin Miller were tireless in their editing support and optimism. Thanks to Christopher Frizzelle for the use of his essay and for his astute suggestions. Thanks to Mariel Povolny, Jeb Lewis, and Linda Mitchell for making music with me.

I honor the work of music therapists whose intensive, creative, and more elaborative therapeutic approach is highly valuable with patients who experience psychosis, and other mental health conditions as well as numerous other health-related issues. I particularly would like to thank Joanne Loewy, and John Mondanaro, of Beth Israel Hospital's Louis Armstrong Center.

Many thanks to Dr. Robert Bergman, Diane Grise, Peggy Swenson, and members of the Society for Psychoanalytic Study and Institute, and the Northwest Alliance for Psychoanalytic Study for helping to broaden my theoretical foundation.

Thanks to Dr. Fer and Dr. Salazar, and to Kay Schisler, Sue Sellers, and Paul Ready, and to all the folks who fought, knitted, and fretted for a second chance.

Thanks to the Wagner Society of Northern California and David Möschler for the photographs and for permission to use Cal Pedranti's art.

Thanks to the Partial Hospitalization Program team: Alice Morris, Amy Zachara, Dana Andrus, Niki Lewis, Dr. Becky Bay, Ephrat Gilad, and Rachel Brantley. Thanks are extended to the Jack's Helping Hand Foundation and to Bridget Ready.

I am very appreciative to Rowman & Littlefield and Lexington Books editors Molly White, Amy King, Alison Pavan, and Kasey Beduhn for their editing guidance, patience, and kindness throughout the manuscript drafting process.

This book is dedicated to Frith, Shirley, and Allen.

My gratitude is extended to the following publishers and publications who have given permission to use excerpts from previously published work:

My gratitude to *The Stranger* for permission to use excerpts from:

Frizzelle, C. (2012, August 12). The woman in 606. *The Stranger.* Retrieved from www.thestranger.com Copyright The Stranger. Reprinted with permission of The Stranger.

Thank you to Satchnote Press for permission to use excerpts from:

Ready, T. (2013). The listening room, In J. Mondanaro & G. Sara (Eds), *Music and medicine: Integrative models in pain medicine.* New York, NY: Satchnote Press. Copyright Satchnote Press. Reprinted with permission of Satchnote Press.

Thanks to Sage Publications Inc.'s permission to use excerpts from the following material:

Ready, T. (2011). Containment and communication through musical preference, *Music and Medicine, 10*(3), 246–257.
Ready, T. (2010). Music as language, *American Journal of Hospice and Palliative Medicine, 27*(1), 7–15.

Thanks to Rowman & Littlefield Publishers for permission to excerpt from:

Ready, T. (2014). Sounding home. In M. O'Loughlin & M. Charles (Eds), *Fragments of trauma and the social production of suffering*. Lanham, MD: Rowman & Littlefield Publishers.

Thanks to Karnac Press for permission to quote from the following publications:

Bion, W. R. (1963). *Elements of psycho-analysis*. London, UK: Karnac.
Bion, W. R. (1984). *Second thoughts: Selected papers on psychoanalysis* New York, NY: Karnac.
Bion, W. R. (1984b). *Learning from experience*. London, UK: Karnac.
Bion, W. R. (1990). *Brazilian lectures*. New York: Karnac.
Bion, W. R. (1992). *Cogitations*. London, UK: Karnac (Original work pubished in 1957).
Grotstein, J. S. (2007). *A beam of intense darkness*. London, UK: Karnac.

Thanks to the Wagner Society of Northern California for permission to use Cal Pedranti's painting *Wielach so hell und Hehr, Gluhender Glanz*. Additional thanks are extended to Joan Lam for her photograph of the painting.

Chapter 1

Introduction

I first learned from my infant nephew, Jack, that music is capable of facilitating the expression of affect and the scaffolding of complex, otherwise ineffable emotions. Music served an auxiliary mothering function for Jack. He would point to the stereo and make a roaring sound until an older sibling would select John Lennon's (1971) "Imagine." Once the first minor chords sounded, Jack would sway and pat one small hand on the rail of his walker.

Jack was never able to speak due to a tenacious, recurring tumor on his brain stem diagnosed when he was twelve weeks old. He underwent contiguous surgeries and cutting-edge treatments. During the course of numerous, extended hospitalizations, music became Jack's language. Sometimes he selected TV cartoon tunes; sometimes he chose lullabies. He might have picked his beloved "Imagine" (Lennon, 1971), for its simple chord progression, or for the reassuring cadence of Lennon's voice, or because his parents or siblings responded positively to the song. Perhaps "Imagine" relieved pain or provided a distraction, or it was a transitional object linked in Jack's unconscious mind to his mother's voice.

"Imagine" played at Jack's memorial service six months after his third birthday. The song united congregants under the vaulted ceilings of the church. It created a second virtual structure within which we could bear the changing weathers of grief. "Imagine" invited us to surrender and embrace the uncertainty of the moment by conjuring a world of peace, harmony, and compassion. The song was more mystical than the practical sermon penned by the priest, who admitted, "My words have been upstaged by an infant." "Imagine" provided solace for Jack's family, friends, and caretakers. Was it the infant's voice speaking, in advance, to the need in us for one another and for a comforting object to hold when Jack was gone? Fifteen years later, that song still recalls the child's image, and, sometimes with it, intimations of joy.

Jack was my primary inspiration for considering music as an adjunct therapeutic tool with patients for whom language had been obstructed. My second muse was my uncle. When he gradually lost language to dementia, opera music opened between us as an alternative portal of expression. At age seventeen, my uncle had experienced a sort of "Deus ex machina" facilitated by music while quarantined in a tuberculosis sanatorium in Los Angeles. In the throes of high fever, he heard Wagner's, "Tannhaüser" sung by Laruitz Melchior (Stuart, 2015) on a 1941 radio broadcast. It was the music, he claimed, that saved him from the brink of death. Thereafter, he devoted his life to painting scenes from operas. I remember sitting with him for long hours in his nineteenth-century bohemian parlor listening to opera highlights. He narrated the libretto and acted out each scene. If I fell asleep during an opera performance I was briefly banished from his home. "Are you a heathen?" he would ask. My musical taste leaned toward jazz, folk, and rock music.

From both my uncle's and Jack's passion for music, I learned that in times of challenge or crisis, complex emotional states may be better contained by crashing opera overtures, or melancholy rock ballads than by language alone. Music carries resonance for humans where language falls short. As a therapist (who had worked for years with homeless youth) I questioned how self-selected music could help establish a portal between a clinician's inner life and a patient's inner life, and how psychoanalytic theory might describe this process. I embarked on a research study and a therapeutic inquiry about using music as an adjunct tool with patients who were experiencing psychosis.

When I first started employing music to help build rapport with patients, I believed European classical music, upon which most empirical studies were based (Juslin & Laukka, 2003; Konecni, 2008), was the key to help patients unlock and express emotions. Likewise, the majority of psychoanalytic texts about music focused on Western classical music. I also anticipated that music without words would provide greater emotional containment for patients. Both these assumptions proved incorrect. A meta-analysis of qualitative research by Silverman (2003) showed that classical music did not prove as effective as popular (or non classical) music in reducing psychotic symptoms.

Another initial oversight was that I did not account for the role of the body as the sensory receptor and mediator of musical containment. Ethnomusicologist Molino (2000) emphasized "rhythmo-affective semantics" in human responses to music: paying attention to the "body, its movements and the fundamental emotions that are associated with them" (p. 170). Molino saw as much merit in studying primitive music and disco as European classical music in order to understand how emotions and music entwine. Rose (2004) elaborated on Bucci's (1985, 1997) descriptions of how non verbal input is encoded and stored in perceptual forms which include kinesthetic, visceral, and sensory impressions such as pictures, sounds, tastes, smells, and feelings. Our aesthetic preferences for music may be obtained, stored, shared, retrieved, and maintained, much like the processes of implicit memory. Thus, Metallica, if that particular genre of music is encoded as consoling, may be more profoundly calming for a person than Yo-Yo Ma's cello renditions of Bach.

With the help of psychoanalytic theory, and bolstered by other music-based research, I hope to illustrate that the same dynamics that animate and compel emotional regulation and attunement in the mother-infant dyad are present and equally potent when working with adult patients in states of intense and ineffable emotional suffering. In addition, music can articulate and symbolize affect and experience in a manner that lets patients share material they may not have consciously processed, but which is mastered within the music or musician, thus allowing them to maintain a sense of dignity and agency in a therapeutic exchange.

Writers and researchers (Darwin, 1871; Patel, 2008; Brandt, Gebrien & Slevic, 2011) have suggested that music may be our first language—beginning with our mother's heartbeat from within the womb. We may learn to attune to her steady modulations, or we may become unsettled by the high pitch of her wavering voice, and her rapid pulse. Music seems to have the potential to reach through to deeper layers of unconscious silence where language may be too complex or threatening (Freud, 1957; Jung, 1977). The *Music in Therapeutic Practice* proposes that listening with patients to their selected music is a highly effective adjunct tool clinicians can employ to connect with patients. Music works especially well with hard-to-reach patients, such as those experiencing psychosis or traumatic re-enactments, many of whom may already, albeit inadvertently, use music as a primary form of self-expression and self-organization.

Consider, for example, Abbey, a twenty-eight-year-old female who was experiencing psychosis related to bipolar disorder, exacerbated by post-traumatic stress disorder (PTSD). She was caught in the throes of a dramatic fragmentation, wherein she could not make sense of her chaotic internal phenomena. Unable to discern whether medical staff were trying to help her or destroy her, Abbey performed her inner conflict by attacking hospital staff. She requested that I download the soundtrack from the Breakfast Club (Forsey, 1985) after attending a music-based process group. We listened to tracks from that album, while she linked the hospital and staff members to characters and scenes from that film. That exercise helped Abbey feel safer. Eventually she dropped the metaphor. Her musical choices shifted to Madonna, and the Eurythmics—80s music that she associated with her early childhood. The music symbolized her relationship with her mother, and symbolized the fantasy structure she maintained to defend against her childhood experiences of neglect and abuse.

We live an era wherein electronic devices that record and play music are considered essential; they reflect our cultures, and sub-cultures and are, thereby, self-defining (Hargreaves & North, 1999; Mickel & Mickel, 2002; Schulkind, Hennis, & Rubin, 1999; Tekman & Hotascu, 2002). Young people, particularly, walk through their daily lives listening to self-selected soundtracks that mediate and memorialize their sensory connections to the world. Thus, a personal music listening device, such as an iPod, can become a symbol for an individual self—we are what we listen to.

In building a case for the use of music in clinical work, I rely on object relations-based notions of containment as expressed by Bion (1993) and Grotstein (1995a, 1995b), including Bion's (1962, 1992) alpha function concepts of "mothering function" and "metabolizing" (Bion, 1967/1984b). The intersubjective relational concept of attunement and the musical basis of the mother-infant dyad are explored through such theorists as Stern (1985), Trevarthen (1984, 1999), Beebe (1986, 1977), and Panksepp (2008). I will consider Winnicott's (1971) notions of potential space and the transitional object. Recent research and theory on the origins and nature of psychosis will also be discussed. I will outline new developments by McGorry and Yung (2003), among others, in the staging of psychosis with particular emphasis on the urgent nature of building therapeutic rapport with early psychosis patients. These researchers have defined early psychosis as a crucial window of opportunity to engage young patients in treatment.

I will bring a synthesis of theories to life through several psychoanalytic-based case studies focused on music listening research, conducted with patients experiencing early psychosis. I will draw from individual sessions and weekly groups that I facilitated with patients in both an acute psychiatric hospital and a partial hospitalization program setting.

Besides creating a portal for communication, I believe that music can help a practitioner develop flexibility, openness, and cultural sensitivity. Overall, music can be useful for patients of all ages who suffer through stress, intense symptoms, and isolation. Patients' families can learn to use music as a coping or communication skill. We will discuss instances when music may negatively impact a therapeutic situation or when music is inappropriate as an adjunct tool.

Listening to music with patients is a combined implicit and explicit process much like the co-creation of a narrative springing from found language. Throughout this book I refer to an iPod that contains the self-selected music of hundreds of patients who attended individual and group sessions over the course of eight years. The iPod stored and memorialized stories of patients joining with a clinical therapist. If patients returned to the hospital they could find a record of themselves as having existed in the space that their beloved stored songs occupied. Otherwise the hospital was a place of disappearances and erasures, of both patients and staff. Most patients stayed for under ten days, and there was high staff turnover.

One young bipolar patient, Valerie, who liked to sing karaoke-style, along with Joss Stone's songs when she was distressed, had remained out of the hospital and stable for eighteen months. Valerie returned to the hospital in a bout of intense mania that led to a psychotic episode. What had precipitated Valerie's psychosis this time was the shock of her husband's plans to serve her divorce papers. Valerie was attending music group when she received the legal documents. She sat in tearful shock, with the legal letter folded closed in her lap. I selected one of Valerie's favorite Joss Stone songs. Valerie burst into "Right to Be Wrong" (Stone, Child & Wright, 2004). Her anger and anguish, contained within Stone's simple melody, was carried, calmed, and called out to the room of listeners.

Chapter 2

Metaphors of Music

A Literature Review

An urgent morning announcement over the hospital loudspeaker called available staff to the acute unit. The first staff member on site discovered the sewer system on the brink of backing up. The rest of our staff devised a hurried plan to rally patients, many of whom were experiencing acute psychosis, out of their rooms and into the public dayroom. We secretly coded this manic maneuver a fire drill. We were worried mayhem would ensue if the patients noticed sinks and toilets overflowing. In the intensive care area, an agitated patient pounded on the door, yelling, "Mount St Helens."

I took a detour to my office to fetch the iPod and portable speaker. Then I returned to the dayroom, calling out "group time." Patients were restless, cranky, and confused; many of them still wore pajamas.

"Let's start with some music we listened to yesterday," I said. Every weekday afternoon I facilitated a group focused around music on the acute unit. Several times per week I downloaded patient requests for particular songs. The iPod held a stored history of about three thousand patient-selected songs. On that morning, I started with Otis Redding's "(Sittin' on The Dock of the Bay" (Redding & Cropper, 1968, Track 1), followed by Journey's "Don't Stop Believin" (Cain, Perry, & Schon, 1981, Track 2). Next I switched to a song patients often requested for its calming effect: Israel Kamakawiwo'ole's version of "Somewhere Over the Rainbow" (Arlen & Harburg, 1939, Track 10).

During the pantomime fire drill, twenty-nine patients packed the dayroom listening intently to the same songs; some of them joined in impromptu karaoke. The young man who had been pounding on the quiet room door sat down and wept. All of us—distressed patients and staff alike—were calmed by the music, joined in the potential space (Winnicott, 1971) music had framed for us. Fortunately, the pipes did not flood the unit, although we were prepared for that emergency. This scene illustrated symbolically and literally the distinct benefits of music as an adjunct treatment modality, at times and in moments, when perceived danger threatens to arise and overwhelm us.

Beginning 1.8 million years ago, humans discovered that coping together through musical expression was a far better survival strategy than being solitary. Our primal urge to connect and attach in relationships is the same urge that inspired the early invention of music (Dissanayake, 2000, 2009). Music's therapeutic potential to calm, animate, comfort, organize, and synchronize humans has been lauded in modern times (Sacks, 2007, xii).

Sharing music as we did during the averted hospital plumbing crisis helped calm both patients and staff during an hour of uncertainty. Kramer (2004) observed that both the cyclic and repetitive nature of music, including the constant beat to which listeners can entrain (synchronize) their bodily motion, as well as deviations from expected regularities, are part of what makes music calming. Vital functions of the body such as heart rate, muscular activity, and respiration can fall into synchrony with music (Rose, 2004; Harrer & Harrer, 1977).

The history of employing music for curative properties hails back to the Greeks. Hippocrates and Plato advocated for the healing function of music (in Storr, 1992). The Adyghs of the North Caucasus have used music for centuries as a means of treating the body and soul in addressing small pox, bullet wounds, snakebites, and bone trauma (Sokolova, 2006). Music therapy has evolved into its own esteemed discipline that addresses the multiple therapeutic uses for music in hospitals, hospices, prisons, community centers, schools, and other settings. I deeply honor the expertise and scope of music therapists. I have been inspired by the work of Joanne Loewy, who developed the technique of song sensitization to work elaboratively with familiar music, as well as Dileo and Parker who have used familiar songs in working with hospice patients. Although I am interested in working with patient's familiar music, this is not a music therapy book.

The *Music in Therapeutic Practice* is intended to prompt clinical therapists, particularly clinicians who take inspiration from psychoanalytic and psychodynamic theoretical models, to incorporate music as a means of building strong, immediate rapport with difficult-to-reach patients. In the hard-to-reach category, I include late adolescent and young adult patients struggling with early psychosis, emerging and chronic mood disorder patients, patients experiencing PTSD, borderline personality disorder patients, alexithymic patients, and patients who struggle with strong suicidal thoughts and urges.

Music is a useful adjunct tool for establishing rapport and for guiding the rhythm of attunement essential to the therapeutic process. Music does not replace or subvert the need for talk therapy; however, music may better assist in the initial expression of painful psychological material that may be otherwise unspeakable.

Nagel (2013) warns against reductionism and tidy explanations when clinicians discuss the power of music. I would add a counter caution against over-intellectualizing the therapeutic aspects of music, which may be implicit and visceral in nature. A Hawaiian lullaby strummed on a ukulele by Iz may parallel a Beethoven symphony in its potential to contain and organize a listener's inner life.

The significance of music as a source of linking, communication, and providing psychic content useful for treatment has been well explored within the psychoanalytic and psychodynamic tradition (Nagel, 2013; Rose, 2004; Lachman, 2001; Kohut, 1972). Reik (1953) observed mid-century that "music is the language of psychic reality." His observation came at a time when art was considered by psychologists to relate to sublimation, vicarious means of conflict resolution, and affect abreaction (Lachman, 2001).

Freud (1897, 1914) was a consumer of opera, at least opera's visual and verbal aspects (in Nagel, 2013), even though he garnered scarce pleasure from music. He remained wary of music as a primary vehicle for delivering unconscious material for interpretation, because he could not articulate the mechanism by which music impacted the psyche; he preferred the exploration of dreams, and the more aesthetically pleasing potency of other arts such as literature and sculpture (Freud, 1914). Nagel (2013) refers to Cheshire's (1996) essay on Freud's relationship to music to support speculation that despite Freud's preferences, he understood music offered emotional containment and restraint.

Contemporaries of Freud were more curious about the affective, symbolic, and metaphoric potential of music. Max Graf (1942), a musicologist and historian, utilized Freud's topographic model to explain music's function as a portal to the unconscious (Abrams in Nigel, 2013). Ehrzenweig (1975) eventually pronounced language and music—which he referred to as a symbolic language—as legitimate paths to unconscious mental processes (in Nagel, 2013).

Nagel (2013) meticulously traces where "oral and aural roads" converge and diverge throughout the relatively brief history of modern psychology (p. 19). Noy (1967) perceived musical structure as being similar to dreams, daydreams, or jokes, thus capable of being psychoanalyzed to uncover latent content (p. 45). The majority of psychoanalytic writing on music pertains to theorists analyzing the inner worlds of composers or musicians, or theorists/ psychoanalysts who are classical or jazz musicians, exploring how psychic material is represented in formal pieces of music.

Another area of psychodynamic focus has been on the musical dimensions of attachment. Beginning with a mother's heartbeat, music is at the center of early attunement—forging powerful connections between infant and mother (Beebe in Lachman, 2001). Rhythm, melody, tone, and repetition are the elements that establish the potency and significance of early affective experience and associations (Kohut and Levarie, 1950). An infant might associate a mother's voice with oral gratification, and her lullaby with sweet satiation after feeding. On the other hand, a highly anxious or disorganized mother's voice could signify danger to an infant. In that case, silence or withdrawal might offer an infant ambivalent comfort.

Early musical interactions, and music, tend to be processed in the right hemisphere of both mother and infant. The right hemisphere is the region that governs emotional, non-verbal aspects of speech such as facial expression and prosody (Feder, 1993). We are born oriented to move from shared pulse and heartbeat toward rhythmically coordinated interpersonal interactions (Lachman, 2001). Patel (2008) suggested that maternal singing was probably an adaptive function, so that mothers could put their children down, while they continued to hold them with the touch of song while foraging for, or preparing, food. Future research might show that an infant's autonomic reflexes are set to the pace and homeostatic points of the mother's voice and the rhythms of her body.

Babies can learn to match pitch, intensity, melodic contour, and the rhythmic structure of a mother's song (Emde, 1983). The rhythmic coordination between infant and caregivers in the form of coos, squawks, and gestures has been christened by Trevarthen (2005) as "communicative musicality." These sounds are the basis of emotions and the means for modifying emotions. Beebee and Stern (1977) experimented with using rhythm, tone, and volume of vocalization to modulate an infant's level of distress and arousal. Stern (1995) found that aside from being the scaffold for affect, early rhythms may be a source of both familiarity and novelty. Nagel (2013) observed early "aural experiences" and non-verbal communications set the foundation for object constancy, object loss, social interactions, and self-definition.

Information about infant communication can be valuable to a clinician when sitting across from an alexithymic or an early psychosis patient if we consider that emotional states exchanged between mother and infant can be shared between therapist and patient (Rosenbaum & Harder, 2007). Traditionally, a therapeutic alliance has been described as being built on the connections of discrete behavioral states such as joy, fear, sadness/distress, anger, disgust, shame, and interest/surprise (Ekman, 1992; Emde, 1988; Tomkins, 1962). Affect states may be expressed through language, or through sounds, noises, simple utterances, and body language, all of which underlie the flow of communication between therapist and patient (Garfield, 2001). This non-verbal stream of messages is what Kohut (1957) referred to when he advised clinicians to listen to "the music that lies behind meaningful words" (p. 243).

To emphasize that the music of both patient and therapist are of equal importance I turn first to Bion (1967/1984b), who suggested that the very music of a practitioner's voice impacts the therapeutic alliance. Psychoanalyst and musician Knoblauch (2000) used the term "musical edge" to describe how the process contours of therapy (volume, tone, tempo, rhythm. and turn taking) emerged in dialogue. Knoblaugh (2000) insisted that a psychotherapist be receptive to all levels of communication—"intimate, primitive, poetic, or musical edges"—so that there was "richer range of meaning and affect available" (p. 825). This same attentiveness is necessary when listening to music with patients. A therapist needs to sustain a state of openness—abiding as Bion (1967/1984b) advised in a state of suspended memory and desire.

Reik (1953) linked the analytic state of mind with musical listening, by comparing the analyst's unconscious to a "musical instrument" (Nagel, 2013; Barale and Minazzi, 2008). He did not posit—although it would have been a reasonable leap—that the unconscious of the patient is another musical instrument. Lachman (2001) and Knoblauch (2000, 2005) made overtures to the importance of co-creation between therapist and patient. Lachman (2001) observed that, when listening to patients' associations, therapists' accompanying rhythms would alter, as each person molded his rhythm to the rhythm of the other. Lachman (2001) predicted that the shared repertoire of rhythms could be coordinated and syncopated (p. 173).

Feder (2004) referred in a presentation to music as a "simulacrum of mental life" (in Nagel, 2013; Barale & Minazzi, 2008). He saw music as being able to illuminate elements of the underlying structures of the mind (Feder in Nagel, 2013). Numerous psychoanalytic and neurobiological theorists have proposed that music stimulates emotions and that there are multiple, simultaneous layered sounds that are constantly represented and processed in the mind. These dynamic processes can occur in a manner that is both intrapsychic and relational (Noy, 1993; Feder, 1993, 2004; Nagel, 2007, 2008, 2008b, 2010, 2013, Lachman, 2001). Langer (2009/1942, 1953) had previously posited that music was akin to the preverbal structure of a person's life. Drawing on the words and work of a myriad of theorists, this writer contends that, if a person's beloved music reflects aspects of his inner life, then sharing music with a therapist can potentially help that patient to synchronize, expand, or enrich his awareness of that inner life.

Another powerful pull in music, Lachman (2001) referred to as a striving toward self-assertion, self-articulation and toward defining oneself uniquely. The act of listening to music with patients—especially adolescents or young adults—can facilitate greater experimentation and self-exploration during therapeutic sessions. Listening to rap, hip-hop, or electronic music can offer a safe frame within which young people learn to master the conflicts between internal rhythms and the chaotic pulse and pull of a modern high-tech world. Adolescents, and adults, perceive popular music stars as mentors or visionaries who can articulate felt emotions that the listener cannot yet express. Musicians may offer alternative paths to the adult world, and provide a "new holding environment" or transitional space created by the listener. An adolescent, or young adult, can collect and own his own "transitional tunes" (McDonald, 1970) while gaining omnipotence and mastery in the process of establishing his own identity (Rosenblum, Daniolos, Kass, & Marin, 1999).

Psychotherapy involves two people playing, according to Winnicott (1958). Music can become part of a co-constructed frame within which therapist and patient can play; it is also a vehicle for expression, and an object for releasing and investing emotions. Young people, and cautious adults, can both reveal and keep secret their most private thoughts when they are expressed through music.

Noy (1993) believed that the same qualities of music that other theorists have linked to early attunement, as well as the creative displacements and manipulations inherent in music, may allow listeners to integrate and achieve multiple levels of complex mental polyphony. I believe that the coordinated call and response between a patient and a therapist, mediated by music, helps allow for more complex ways of organizing and containing affect and experience for the patient, and moreover, for both participants.

In considering how shared music might offer an organizing and scaffolding function for both therapist and patient, Winnicott's (1953) concept of the transitional object is useful. From the infant's point of view, the transitional object is his creation, and simultaneously, it exists there in the environment for the infant's use. From the mother's point of view, the object soothes the infants' anxiety (as well as her own) at departure times. McDonald (1970) developed this concept into the idea of a "transitional tune" in which a piece of music, such as a lullaby, can provide a shared comforting experience by filling the space between separation and return. The song "Imagine" was a shared transitional tune between my nephew, Jack, and his mother. Jack created "Imagine" each time he pointed at the stereo. His mother cherished the musical affirmation of hope, even after the child had died, as if through the vehicle of the song he returned again. In a theoretical mechanical sense, "Imagine" was invested with narcissistic and object libido (McDonald, 1970).

Acquiring and consciously accessing transitional tunes could help patients to learn and practice impulse control, affect regulation, neutralization, and sublimation. These skills could become elaborated by adding other songs to the shared repertoire, gradually encouraging more layered and complex pieces of shared music, or a give-and-take of therapist and patient music.

I have presented theoretical and philosophical material to support the use of music as an adjunct therapeutic tool beneficial to a variety of patients. What I have not yet discussed is how trauma complicates the process of establishing rapport and connection with patients. In *The Cognitive Psychotherapy of Schizophrenia*, Kingdon and Turkington (2005) proposed trauma as one of the four predispositions that can lead to psychosis. Morrison and colleagues (2003) go so far as to suggest that PTSD and psychosis may lie on a spectrum of responses to trauma. For patients with psychosis as well as other diagnoses that may have origins in trauma—such as bipolar disorder, PTSD, or borderline personality disorder—developing trusting relationships with therapists and professionals can be a dangerous prospect. To connect opens the potential for annihilation (the breakdown of the self) and abandonment with a concurrent loss of ability to modulate thought and feeling through language, life can seem chaotic and menacing to these patients (Leite, 2003).

Music may be better equipped to address painful emotional memories that are encoded, organized, and stored in a non-verbal manner through kinesthetic and visceral forms as well as through other sensory representations (Bucci, 1985, 1997, in Rose, 2004). With trauma, a rift between the observing and experiencing aspects of the ego occurs (Fromm, 1965). Music is a window into traumatic experiences that are split off or dissociated into physical or psychological symptoms (Knoblauch, 2000) Listening to music with a therapist can be an ideal vehicle for organizing, or at least containing emotions, and eventually processing them and explicitly integrating them with other experiences in a relational setting (van der Kolk, McFarlane, & Weisaeth, 1996). Music supports an optimal working relationship between the observing and experiencing aspects of the ego to help with positively toned affect regulation (Rose, 2004, p. 129).

Psychoanalytic theorists and neurobiologists converge on the notion that the most severe forms of psychopathology may be caused by a serious developmental or environmental trauma that has a particularly impact on people who are highly sensitive to environmental stimuli (Bion, 1957/1984d; Schore, 2002; Schore, 1994; van der Kolk, Roth, Pelcovitz, Sunday, & Spinazzola, 2005). Without a sufficient caregiver or environmental mediator in breaking down experiences, sensations, and emotions, and digesting them through the help of imagination, fantasy, illusion, and symbolization, infants can become overwhelmed beyond their nervous system's threshold capacity (McEwen, 2003; Mulvihill, 2005, Nijenhuis, 2004). Grotstein's (1995a) term "orphans of the 'Real'" describes "patients who have awakened too early and too painfully from the protection of the passive stimulus barrier of the perinatal period or from the active stimulus barrier that normally issues from bonding and attachment" (p. 2).

Music may be particularly useful for patients with severe mental health issues. Studies have demonstrated the relaxing and organizing effect of music on schizophrenic patients (Glickson & Cohen, 2000; Neilzen & Cesarec, 1981). In addition, music-based interventions diminish negative symptoms (anhedonia, anxiety) and improve interpersonal contact for inpatient schizophrenic patients.

Music can help define a safe container, breaking language down into beta elements of rhythm (Bion, 1950, 1967/1984b). Listening to music with a therapist can offer a positive experience of projective identification wherein the person is contained simultaneously by the prosody of pre-verbal rhythms, while sitting with a person who can share, and help metabolize, the emotional experience of listening.

With teenagers and young adults who might be hesitant to directly discuss feelings, music may be especially helpful as an adjunct therapeutic tool (Rosenblum et al., 1999). The tasks of adolescence involve decathecting from early object ties to strive toward autonomy and a newly consolidated sense of self. Adolescents wrangle with such issues as letting go grief and perceived abandonment. They oscillate between progression and regression, and autonomy and independence (Blos, 1962). Rather than adding to increased feelings of isolation and doubt, music provides settings within which unconscious conflicts may be played out and resolved through displacement (Rosenblum et al., 1999).

The rhythms and repetitive tempos of modern songs may be more aligned or more unconsciously recognizable and accessible than classical music for young people. Songs by Beyoncé, Daft Punk, or Lady Gaga encourage social participation and body awareness. Music can allow for an "immediate visceral collaboration with the adolescent patient" (Rosenblum et al., 1999).

In working with both adolescents and adults, I concur with Rose (2004) that music allows a constantly shifting balance to occur between therapist and patient. What's more, the music itself can hold the role of a witnessing presence (Rose, 1996) for patients' emotional experiences, including trauma. Music is an entity capable of watching and listening. It may not always be possible to have constant intersubjective equality, but music may honor the aspiration for what Rose (2004) called an "asymmetrical working partnership." Ideally, interactions between therapist and patient mediated by music would involve various layers and inflections. These interactions could be an open improvisation, full of match and mismatch, and harmonization and counterbalance (Keil and Feld, 1994). With music, meanings might unfold and emerge that are a surprise to either party, or be connected indivisibly to both (Rose, 2004).

Because the process of infant attachment is so closely attuned to musical processes writers have referred to music as our first language or as the language of emotions. Nagel (2013) warned against such facile comparisons. She conceptualized music and psychoanalysis as representations of emotional life. In considering music as a source of "pertinent psychoanalytic data," she recommends a nuanced and less reductionist approach. At the same time, Nagel calls for the necessity of psychoanalysts to take a leading role in addressing important community and social problems (Twemlow in Nagel, 2013).

We began this chapter exploring the power of music to help foster a sense of attunement within the temporary community of a psychiatric hospital. An environmental threat—the specter of sewage resurfacing—had symbolic implications if viewed as the environment in its own state of hallucinosis (Bion). Sewage could symbolize patients' unprocessed impressions, trauma, and other beta (or raw emotional) material—re-emerging as voices, hallucinations, and sense-based projections. All of that unconscious material threatened to spill out and overwhelm the plumbing system. There was a palpable, rising dread among staff and patients. In the midst of a chaotic situation, the hospital staff and the patients were soothed when listening to and attuning to familiar music. Staff was better able to contain the chaos and anxiety of the patients by processing their own fear, anger, and dread of the unknown collectively with music.

The ongoing relevance of psychoanalysis in a fast-paced world will be tied to our ability to adapt to technologically sophisticated and fragmenting social structures. Popular music may lack the depth, nuance, and complexity of classical music, but it is our best, most accessible portal to some patients' inner worlds. Any form of music that can help inspire people who are suffering from mental health issues to reconnect and build rapport with a therapist is worth considering. Even heavy metal could be useful in mental health recovery. The themes and theories introduced here will be explored through case studies and vignettes, and synthesized in the final chapter.

Chapter 3

Music and Bonding

Orlando, who is not yet twenty years old, arrived for a meeting with his parents. Orlando rested his head on the table while his parents asked questions. When will he return to normal? Where is his motivation? Why does he hide in his room all day? Orlando's mother described changes in her son's behaviors. Months ago he had sold snacks at a sports stadium. He made good tips. He was gregarious. Then suddenly, his normal routine abruptly ended.

Orlando didn't remember how events unfolded. Just before things began to reel out of control, he experienced himself as being socially adept and fluid in contrast to his usual awkwardness. His mind moved so fast, he could quickly synthesize and draw together disparate topics, and turn clever phrases at will. There had been greater ease until the final catastrophe of being locked inside a psychiatric hospital. Afterwards, Orlando felt himself moving in slow motion. People stared. Were they laughing at the blank expressions on his face? When he looked in the mirror he saw an alien. He could no longer keep up with friends' quick banter. He felt socially self-conscious.

Part of Orlando's discomfort involved voices urging him toward senseless activities such as tearing up old photographs. One voice sounded like his mother, calling him "monster" as she did repeatedly at the height of a manic episode. Her words joined the chorus of voices echoing inside him. Other voices ordered him to look at his own distorted face in the mirror.

Orlando refused to meet with outside providers, or to follow a medical protocol. He ended up circling through psychiatric hospitals and jail several times. He became suspicious that every clinical professional wanted to" incarcerate" him. When Orlando listened to ambient music on his iPhone, the voices quieted down. "They slipped under the piano keys," he said. "I could breathe." Our work together involved bringing music into the shared social space of a dyad or group, to build trust with Orlando while listening to music.

From the moment Orlando walked through the hospital doors, he had a fairly secure and active attachment to music as an object and as a mediator of his emotions and symptoms. He used rhythm, tone, volume, and vocalization (Beebe & Stern, 1977) to modulate his distress and arousal, although if asked directly he would have denied any conscious intent to manage affects. My participation in his ongoing relationship to music allowed me to expediently join in his process of emotional mediation as a witness, a participant observer, and as an auxiliary ego for Orlando (Fromm-Reichman, 1959).

Panksepp and Trevarthen (2009) referred to the brain as an "organ of intersubjective collaboration with systems of emotional regulation that are fundamentally musical." I hope to illustrate in this chapter with the help of intersubjective/relational theory that the same dynamics that compel emotional regulation and attunement in the mother-infant dyad are equally essential when working with adult patients in states of intense, overwhelming emotional suffering. Employing self-selected music as an alternative portal—or what Nagel (2013) referred to as an "aural road"—to unconscious material can also help psychotherapists attend to transference and countertransference amidst challenging clinical work. Music is appealing for humans, according to Panksepp (2008), because of the activation of social emotional processes, some of which, like mother-infant bonding, are addictive. These addictive aspects of music may be beneficial in fostering a socially bonded life, within which a patient can gradually learn to attach to an intimate other (Panksepp, 2008). I will discuss the negative aspects of music's addictive features and how music may even stimulate addictive cravings later in this chapter.

An awareness of self is an emergent property of the mind appearing in the first half year of life: an emerging sense of self includes an awareness of others (Stern, 1985). Early disturbances in affect and attunement while a child is undergoing this emerging sense of self and other can have dire consequences. Distortions of reality, splits, and fragmentations in the experiencing and recognizing of basic emotions are possible consequences, so is an inhibited ability to experience pleasure (Stern, 1985).

Clinicians who are working with patients who are difficult to engage because of various obstructions such as those noted above may find music useful in building rapport. Music can also help clinicians connect with patients experiencing traumatic re-enactments, acute psychotic episodes, and even issues of diverse languages and culture (which I will discuss in chapter 4). There are particular benefits intrinsic to music that could make it valuable to clinicians working in community settings, in private practice, and in hospitals.

Music helped Orlando allay his own anxieties, and learn to cope with his parents' anxieties about the unknown. Orlando's family encouraged him to take steps toward launching; however, the more his parents pushed, the more his sense of shame about falling behind and feeling socially outcast intensified. We used music to explore ideas about the future, modulating distress through familiar music selections while we discussed options. He wanted to enroll in nursing school, but he dreaded opening the anatomy textbook he had purchased before his recent psychotic episode.

During our work together, Orlando came to understand that his mother's voice was particularly disconcerting to him, unless he concurrently listened to ambient or reggae music or took breaks from conversations. Music helped facilitate this self-awareness both individually and in the context of small groups. For Orlando, the steady voice of Bob Marley provided perfect counterpoint to the dissonance of his mother's anxiety. It was a concrete realization of the validity of how high expressed emotions (EE) (Hooley & Campbell, 2002; Hooley & Gotlib, 2000; Leff & Vaughn, 1985), marked by criticism, hostility, and emotional overinvolvement, can be detrimental to people struggling with psychosis who may well be hypersensitive to their environments (Grotstein, 1995a). For Orlando, the sting of shrillness was soothed by Marley's steady, gentle repetitive voice.

Another nineteen-year-old patient, Hannah, arrived involuntarily at the hospital after claiming she had planted bombs throughout her parents' house. Several days after her admission, her parents confessed that they were pondering plans to relocate Hannah to a semi-independent housing complex. In a sense, her parents had been "planting bombs" of imminent change through secretive planning about deconstructing her family (Ready, 2011). Hannah chose the emotionally detached and cynical lyrics of Suzanne Vega to help her come to terms with an impending loss of her home and her independence.

Hannah had unraveled into a psychotic episode in anticipation of the trauma of abandonment. Music helped Hannah reconnect to a sense of self and to take steps to reconstruct that self to prepare for an imminent change. Hannah explored her Asian American heritage, her romantic history, and her relationship with her father while we listened to the melodies and lyrics of various songs. The other pieces of music she selected (Alice in Chains, Lady Gaga, Celine Dion) were communications about the process of re-ordering her inner life and making sense of collapsed chapters of childhood and early adult experiences. Hannah communicated essential information, embedded in self-selected songs that helped shape her treatment. We focused on her wish to live in an urban apartment inspired by Vega's Manhattan cafés and Brooklyn brownstone ballads.

Like Hannah, many patients arrive in an acute psychiatric hospital after having lost connection to their inner lives; however, these patients may still communicate fragments of their untethered inner lives to others (Ready, 2011). Their transference messages arrive encoded in psychosis to be translated, much like Hannah's "bombs." Philosopher of mind and art Susan Langer (1953) observed that the inner life has similar properties to music: similar patterns of motion and rest, tension and release, agreement and disagreement, as well as preparation, fulfillment, excitation, repetitions, variations and sudden changes. Thus the patterns of inner life may be better expressed through the vehicle of music.

Therapeutic rapport with acute adult patients who are consciously or inadvertently conveying symbolic or metaphoric, sometimes nonverbal, information may be facilitated by understanding the dynamics of the incremental and melodic rhythmic co-creativity that exists between mother and child. Trevarthen (2005) based the dynamics of "communicative musicality" on the elements of pulse, quality, and narrative. Pulse referred to the regular succession of discrete behavioral events (gestures and sounds) through time that occurred in conversation (Malloch, 2000).

When a clinical therapist listens to music with an adult or young person, the same bi-directional dynamics that animate the mother-infant bond are at play. This musical dialogue may translate into nods, songs, eye contact, or proximity with patients. One young man with schizophrenia ran his hands through his hair when he was angry. Another patient straightened, and angled the iPod when feeling dread. When Hannah chose a call-and-response song by the rap artist DMX, for example, it was DMX who set in motion the initial call, but it was the clinician who kept the call and response in motion by listening attentively with Hannah. The song was experienced in present tense, enfolded inside the live bi-directional interaction.

The more a clinician can participate in the act of listening with a completely open and unassuming mind (Bion, 1984), the potentially stronger the therapeutic alliance. Beebe noted that young babies show a profound sensitivity to the interactive contingency and authenticity of a communication partner's rhythm of expression and to the sympathy of feelings expressed by gesture and tone of voice (Beebe, 2003; 2006; Beebe & Lachman, 1994). The act of "listening with" a patient to music includes a similar, ongoing intersubjective dialogue. We listen together. There is an "us" who listens. The existence of that "us" can potentially help maintain a sense of safety in the listening experience (Ready, 2011).

The link between therapist and patient, much like the infant-caretaker connection, need not be perfect. A sense of trust and safety can be created through moments of mis-attunement and repair (Winnicott, 1953; Beebe, 2006). This repair, described by infant researchers as a flexible "interactive" process, involves matching, mismatching, and re-matching again (Beebe, 2006; Beebe & Lachman, 1994; Tronick & Cohn, 1989). Rapport is constructed and fine-tuned in the movement back and forth between similarity and difference (Beebe, 2006; Benjamin, 1995; Knoblauch, 2000).

Hannah eventually progressed from the detachment of Vega's songs to the longing for home and transcendence conveyed in Celine Dion's "Vole" (Goldman, 1995). Hannah's musical choices helped me grasp the extent of her anxiety about her parents' abandonment, which we later addressed through music. Attuned responses by clinicians may assist patients who are learning and practicing emotional self-regulation including down regulation of arousal (Beebe, 2006). I mirrored features of Hanna's musical choices back to her to help facilitate awareness about ways she might want to communicate with her parents in the future.

Listening to self-selected music with patients like Hannah can teach us what qualities and rhythm of voice might be most essential in creating a "good enough" fit or a sense of musical attunement with another (Winnicott, 1958), much like being a *participant observer* of containment while sitting together safely contained in a lulling, boat on a calm lake (Sullivan, 1953). Music fills spaces where language has failed; it allows access to what Beebe (2006) termed "implicit and pre-linguistic forms of communicative competency and intersubjectivity."

Elliot was more outwardly oppositional to treatment than Orlando or Hannah; his reactions to listening together to music were lurching and dramatic. Elliot was a thin, waif-like twenty-three-year-old of mixed Russian and British descent. He shifted from disdain and impatience to unexpected moments of openness, wherein he was curious and explorative. Elliot had recently dropped out of Brown University. His parents hoped he would finish his final credits at the University of British Columbia. Instead, Elliot took refuge in the forests of Stanley Park in Vancouver, British Columbia, emerging a few times per week to drive south to his family's home in Bellingham to garner food, cash, and survival supplies. When his father confronted him, he claimed he was preparing for a secret conference with the Pope. His parents urged him to return to taking prescribed psychiatric medications. Elliot refused. Medications ruined his sex drive and made him feel sedated and numb. In a heated argument with his mother over medications, he physically threatened her, which led to involuntary hospitalization.

During his sophomore year of college, Elliot began attending raves, and experimenting with various illicit substances, including ecstasy, acid, and marijuana. Elliot's grades and schoolwork deteriorated. As Elliot became more involved in the rave scene he also became increasingly paranoid about being surveilled by college roommates. Elliot told friends he was having nightly conversations with Dostoyevsky and Einstein. His delusions became more prominent, featuring Elliot as an omniscient intercessor between Earth and God. His family described him as socially awkward. Just before his hospitalization, and after a perceived flirtation in a bar, Elliot kissed a fraternity brother, who promptly beat him up.

Elliot had been previously detained for two weeks at an East Coast psychiatric hospital where he was diagnosed bipolar I with psychotic features. He started a medication regimen that fell apart soon after discharge. Elliot told his family that he wanted to "leave the human race" numerous times due to the loss of his girlfriend. Elliot's stated reason for returning to the hospital was that he had experimented with too many drugs, which re-sparked his bipolar condition. He said, "I started to see a face in a mirror, which would turn into a ghoulish face that I also saw in the wall. That was quite scary." Elliot was hyper-focused on his reflection. He often looked at himself in windows or in the small reflective square of the iPod screen. Locating himself externally seemed less unsettling than being lost inside emotional chaos. He admitted to hearing command voices and experiencing delusions.

Although Elliot agreed to listen to music together as a diversion while in the hospital, he remained suspicious. He glanced briefly through the iPod and then requested Tool, Alice in Chains, Led Zeppelin, Radiohead, and The Rolling Stones. He also mentioned an interest in Beethoven. One of the first songs he picked was "The Patient" from Tool (2001, Track 3). He said, "It reminds me of my adolescence when I was always in a mystical state of mind. Now I monitor my choices." He described experiencing the movement of his shifting consciousness inside Tool's music: "from everyday awareness to being closer to God. This is something divine, a connection to the sublime." Tool had an existential quality for him. "It's evolutionary," he said, "an explanation of a deeper scheme of life, I associate with being in a dream, but I don't want to follow that out too far."

Elliot's passion for Tool's music, with its spiritual edge, symbolized an experimental time of openness in his life. He described his connection to the music in similar fashion to how Tool's bandleader, James Maynard Keenan, described the band's philosophical intentions—to capture the metaphysical, spiritual, and emotional changes occurring in the modern world (Wiederhorn, 1996). Tool's website entrance portal was dubbed the "collective unconscious" (Jung 1953/1966). In the same Jungian vein, the band strove to create archetypal soundscapes, like video game sounds.

From Tool, Elliot switched to Michael Jackson's "Human Nature," (Porcaro & Bettis, 1982, Track 7), which was new music to him. His affect lightened. I noticed the transference; I paid closer attention than usual to the layers of music when Elliot announced, "There are so many layers. I was listening to the chorus, how he laid down and overdubbed the voice on the CD." This was the first significant experience of shared listening. "That was so well done," he said when it ended. "It was a pleasure to listen to."

In the next session, we had a rupture regarding medications. I stepped outside the frame to promote early psychosis treatment protocols (McGorry & Yung, 2003). Elliot became defended and angry. Directly after the mismatch,

Elliot chose Beethoven's (1796–1797, Track 5) "Piano Concerto No. 1 in C, Major Largo." He listened briefly, and then said, "I don't like it. I thought a concerto was one instrument." He said he preferred to listen alone to his own music.

From that point on, Elliot seemed irritated by sounds. He kicked his chair away from the table, leaning back against the wall. Elliot chose a few classical pieces which, much like Rorschach images, were highly emotionally evocative and disturbing. Elliot had strong negative responses (i.e., grimacing, agitation) when listening to classical music. At the same time, he exhibited a strong sensitivity to nuances and variations in musical production (recording quality, dubbing, layering). At the end of the session, Elliot grudgingly chose to reconnect through Israel Kamakawiwo'ole's (Iz) "Somewhere Over the Rainbow" (Arlen & Harburg, 1939, Track 1). He said, "This gives me a rebellious feeling. No more bells and whistles. I just want his pure voice."

Elliot was strobe-like in his participation. Building clinical rapport with him was delicate. He was initially enthusiastic about sharing impressions, but grew tired of the process. Elliot sometimes edited or revised previous responses, such as wanting to clarify that he was no longer attracted to Tool, or to the band's implicit association with raves and mind-altering substances. In these identity revisions, Elliot seemed bent on destroying or undoing links that we had previously established (Bion, 1959/1984a). In a recent qualitative survey of patients with psychosis regarding music-based treatments Solli and Rolvsjord (2015), observed that some patients cherished music that stood outside the realm of illness, stigma, and treatment. The researchers suggested that music might not be an appropriate modality for patients who want to hold a sanctuary for music in their inner lives.

Elliot did not constantly attack, but allowed for brief connections, such as enjoying IZ or Michael Jackson's "Human Nature" (Porcaro & Bettis, 1982, Track 7). Elliot had a keen sensitivity to the perceived dangers of open communication; he moved between attraction to vulnerability and wanting to destroy it in himself and others (Langs, 1983). For a clinician working with Elliot, exploring the public and private personas of the lead singers of Rolling Stones, Radiohead, and Tool, could invite common inquiry into social norms. Listening to music together could also help fine-tune Elliot's awareness of his sensitivity to nuanced elements of tone and intonation, which he could learn to apply when facing challenging social interactions.

Fachner (2010) observed that intense emotions inspired by music can also activate the brain's reward system, and induce drug memories or addictive cravings connected to the altered state within which the music was experienced. Listening to drug-associated-music with a clinician can provide an intersubjective context within which music can be experienced in a new and perhaps more health-sustaining manner.

Working with young adult patients experiencing psychosis can be frustrating: with progress imperceptible at first and then slow and incremental (Rosenbaum & Harder, 2007). Gaining insight into the rhythm of musical exchange with a patient can subsequently help us better attune to musical elements, or "subtle state shifts" in our verbal exchange with these patients as per Knoblauch's (2000) "musical edge." Latency has its own rhythm of silence and speech that we could learn to match.

Several layers of dialogue, with accompanying rhythmic and tonal shifts and embodied transference, happen simultaneously when listening to music with patients. First, the tangible presence of an iPod and portable speaker may offer familiar comfort to patients. Then, there is an ongoing attachment process through musical attunement. Patient and clinician can experience personal and shared affective and physiological responses to music. These responses become folded into the ongoing dialogue, which will include moments of mismatch or dissonance and moments of matching harmony. A clinician may also gain knowledge about the patient's inner world by continuing to mine the patient's music for meanings through reflection and research even after a session is completed. In the next chapter, I will apply several object relations concepts, particularly the theories of Bion, to listening to self-selected music with patients.

Chapter 4

Blue Eyes, Bread, and Water

We will continue to explore how the dynamics of the mother-infant dyad can operate in helping a clinician establish rapport with a patient, using music, to break down raw emotional material into digestible portions. Adults who have not yet experienced having their fears of death—or other intense affects—suffered and detoxified by a maternal figure through reverie and returned in a manner which could be tolerated and integrated into conscious awareness are still in need of such compassionate containment. This was the case with Harika, a young Middle Eastern woman. I could better understand her circumstances by applying Bion's (1962, 1965, 1984, 1992) theories, of container/contained, the alpha function, the origins of psychosis, and the Real or O to her situation. Bion noted that what has not been transformed and symbolized remains in a person as a kind of emptiness or "nameless dread" (Bion, 1962, p. 116).

Bion (1984, 1984b), who worked extensively with psychotic patients, described attunement and emotional regulation processes as a mental digestive process, which he called the alpha function. A mother could convert, through metabolization, raw sensations, impressions, and emotional projections (known as beta) received from her infant. She could then transform these projections (alpha function) into bearable small pieces (1984, 1984b). A mother, breaking beta pieces down into semiotic elements such as language, could help a child experience containment which could help him organize and think about his affective experience (Bion, 1984b, 1992; Bleandonu, 1994). Bion (1984) perceived alpha function as being as essential to therapy as it was to the mother-infant dyad (Bion, 1984). Otherwise, a psychotic person who completed the act of synthesizing words into thoughts, without a protective mediator, might be exposed to dreaded, preferably avoided aspects of himself. Rather than letting sensory impressions enter the mind, the person with psychosis would attack the very building blocks of thought (Grotstein, 1995).

A clinician can gradually help a patient to handle complex emotional experiences, such as fear of annihilation, by participating in moderating the emotions. Thus, the patient does not "become overwhelmed by too much stimulation" (Charles, 2002, p. 121). Music can serve a further containing function, providing a framework for holding the clinician and the therapist during the process of transference and counterstranference. Music has the capacity to enhance the metabolization and the mentalization (Fonagy) process, especially for patients for whom connecting with therapeutic professionals in a hospital or community setting is painful. The patient may experience the personal listening device, or the music playing on that device, as the object that is listening to him (Rose, 1996).

Bion observed that patients experiencing psychosis, rather than converting impressions into thoughts and feelings, would eliminate the impressions through hallucinations, splitting sensory impressions into good and bad components, or projecting uncomfortable thoughts and feelings back out into the environment, including into other people (Bion, 1955/1984c). In order to transform this kind of structure through psychotherapeutic treatment, the patient would need to develop the ability to tolerate frustration/tensions and emotional arousal long enough for processing to occur.

Harika's first three days on the acute unit of the hospital were a re-enactment of a *primitive catastrophe* (Bion, 1957, 1984d; Grotstein, 2007). Harika pushed against walls as if they would open into doorways. She kneeled on a white bath towel engaging in ritual prayers. She refused to wear clothes, to eat or to interact with staff, attacking all links between objects and between the self and objects (Bion, 1957/1984g; 1959/1984a; 1967b). Harika had been a community college exchange student living with an evangelical Christian host family in Idaho. Dramatic differences in beliefs and lifestyles made the match less than ideal for the Muslim girl.

Her host mother announced before leaving for a business trip that Harika needed to cook and to feed the dog. These were servants' tasks in Harika's family of origin. Harika projected split-off negative and paranoid feelings (Klein 1986/1946) on to her host mother, whom she was certain was trying to poison her.

When the host mother returned, she noticed Harika's actions had become more bizarre—Harika took showers at strange hours. She drank only tea, claiming to want a pure and empty stomach. She became increasingly disorganized. On several occasions she left the front door wide open in the middle of the night when she went on excursions. On one of these night flights, Harika ended up in a hospital emergency room. She demanded that the other patients handcuff her. When she became violently agitated, she was placed in restraints. She seemed to abandon her hold on reality, telling hospital staff her name was Sheba, and that she had been born in the seventeenth century.

Harika went back to the ER three times in a week. She refused medications; her bizarre behaviors increased. She arrived at our hospital in a chaotic state; she was non-communicative with flat affect, and appeared to be responding to voices. Her admitting physician gave her a psychosis, NOS diagnosis. The hospital contacted Harika's father, who pinpointed her unraveling to increased stress from her living situation and from failing a class. He planned to travel to the US to accompany her home. The father called Harika a strong-willed perfectionist who had no previous history of psychological treatment. Harika had been experiencing mood shifts that could have been indicative of bipolar disorder (her brother had been diagnosed with bipolar disorder I). It is also true that Harika's responses to involuntary commitment, to medication, and to treatment were intensified by language, culture and belief (Boke, Aker, Alptekin, Sarisoy, & Sahin, 2007; Ozmen et al., 2005). Overall, Harika seemed lost in an impenetrable darkness.

Harika had immersed herself in American culture in Idaho, subject to the daily stress of being an "other" without adequate support. There were few other Muslim students in her school. Although her English language abilities were sophisticated, her deficits in reality testing caused her to misinterpret communications.

Studies of migrants living in unfamiliar cultures have shown that social support, which Harika lacked, has a strong preventative effect for people otherwise vulnerable to psychosis. In a study of psychosis prevalence in the city of Izmir, Turkey, researchers noted that females were 2.5 times more likely to develop psychotic symptoms and were more likely to display positive symptoms (i.e., hallucinations, delusions) than men (Alptekin, Ulas, Akdede, Tümüklü, & Akyardar, 2009, p. 910).

When I first met Harika, she seemed to me a highly creative, poetic mind dwelling in a metaphorical mineshaft. I thought of the poet Sylvia Plath. That association offered a clue that Harika may be someone with heightened sensitivities, unable to synthesize words into thoughts lest she be exposed to a dreaded aspect of herself, or a haunting memory she preferred to avoid. I was curious if music would allow Harika space to tolerate intense feelings and sense impressions to allow her eventually to draw meaning from her experiences, and rebuild a sense of self.

Harika's physician suggested that I wait a week before approaching her to participate in the music listening project. Our first encounter had been quite concrete. She came to one of the music groups I facilitated. She sat next to me and asked to share a bottle of unopened sparkling water. I poured half the bottle's contents into a paper cup. She drank it, then made another request: "Blue eyes," she said, pointing to the iPod. I would like blue eyes."

After several trial and error music selections, I hit upon Frank Sinatra's "Fly Me to the Moon" (Howard, 1954, Track 3). Harika smiled, saying, "Yes this song. I will follow you wherever you go." At the end of the thirty-minute group Harika grabbed my hand and placed it against her left wrist, twice. Our early rapport was built out of gestures, and objects (water and familiar music) that held potential for future resonant communication. Harika offered initial access to her fragmented internal world. We would gradually try to make sense of fragments together inside the container of music.

Harika's request for "blue eyes" turned out to be culturally, as well as intra-psychically, significant. According to a *National Geographic* (Dede, 2010) article, the roots of Turkish pop music "can be traced back to the late 50s and early 60s when Western styles like jazz, and tango . . ." infiltrated popular consciousness. Pioneering Turkish artists were "influenced by Frank Sinatra, Nat King Cole, and jazz and pop standards"(p. 1). "Fly Me to the Moon" (Howard, 1954, Track 3) had also been chosen by Apollo 11 astronauts for the first moon walk—a modern secular prayer to technology (Kossoff, 2009). The urge to transcend was a theme in my work with Harika.

Harika had difficulty sitting through the initial Rorschach assessment. She left the room, to pray in the hallway. The inkblot images had stimulated unprocessed emotions that she evacuated through action (Bion, 1957/1984g). On our third attempt at the Rorschach, Harika asked to have *Baroque Adagios* (Bach, 1717–1723, Track 1; Vivaldi, 1741, Track 8) playing in the background.

Harika was equally suspicious when we started music sessions. She requested that the door be left ajar. She had wrapped a towel around her head, as scarves were not allowed in the hospital. I showed her how to use the iPod. She found it confusing, but attempted to navigate the dial. Harika selected "Fly Me to the Moon" (Howard, 1954, Track 3). She disliked other Sinatra songs.

Next, Harika selected "Pavane Pour Une Infante Defuntè" (Ravel, 1899, Track 1). She switched because it was "sad." Her choice made me wonder whether one of music's adjunct roles would be to help contain painful beta elements of an unresolved grief. Scrolling through artists, she randomly picked spoken word poet Saul Williams (2002, Track 5). She asked what Williams was doing. I attempted to explain spoken word; Harika's attention ebbed and flowed. She seemed to grasp more at the angry tone and breathless pace of Williams' piece than its meanings. She said, "I do and I do not."

Harika mimicked my movements: she pretended to take notes when I took notes in an act of twinship or gestural mirroring (Decety & Chaminade, 2005) as she had with the sparkling water. I offered Harika a legal pad and pen. She wrote: "I do not or not," then turned the pad toward me to read. Satisfied, she took pen in hand again to write:

Calling her name sometimes. Do or do not. I'm calling her name or not! Who is the slammer in his poet? I'm on not do it. I'm cannot find who is she there. Do I wear or not? Do I go to the watch to put in my arm? Or not to it?

When Harika arrived at the hospital, her words seemed disassembled and patched back together with blended syntaxes. She spoke and wrote English in concrete memes of information (Dawkins, 1976). It was unclear whether she was giving form to her feelings or dismantling feelings to push them further away. Harika had difficulty organizing her primary process thinking into syntax while also operating in a second language. The language translation process seemed to parallel the psychological task inherent in the alpha work of allowing emotions and thoughts to link. In our listening sessions, Harika offered beta elements of language such as "I'm on not do it." She used songs with strong affect as the pool from which to gather her beta material. She grabbed at concrete objects (my watch) and words as objects (slammer, angel). Words shifted and rearranged in her mind, perhaps in the same fluid way she perceived sounds and images changing. She also seemed to be asking indirectly, and on another level simultaneously, if what she saw and heard was real. The sessions were exhausting. Even writing about them now, years later, is difficult as if I am again lost in the murky shadows with Harika.

Harika chose Bach's (1717–1723, Disc 2: Track 1) "Air on a G String" for our second session. She listened briefly, then said it made her more tired. The music was orderly, and formal. At her prompting, I changed to: "Pavanne Pour Une Infante Defuntè" (Ravel, 1899, Track 1). This time she referred to the song as "peaceful," as if we had already begun to sift through grief's wreckage. After two more Ravel pieces, she closed her eyes. "I would be better with the Qur'an," she said. I agreed to find one.

She asked me to choose another song. I selected John Prine's (1971, Track 4) "Angel from Montgomery," mainly for the "angel" which had been the dominant image Harika reported seeing in the Rorschach inkblots, and for the song's primary affect of longing. Harika asked about the meaning. I described "Angel from Montgomery" as an escape fantasy the song's narrator revisited when her world became heavy or dull. Harika wanted to talk about angels and angel lands. She wrote:

Where we go I did not see/But they tried to change, which we cannot see at all/ We cannot see the fate that can only training/ourselves and people around us/I hope so it will and very wisely and mercifully. What can I change?

I read aloud, by her request, the words she had written. The word "angel" was a link and a distortion between us. What did it mean? Did angels and longing offer a doorway into Harika's inner life? A memory? Was she linking or attacking bringing words into meaningful relationships? Harika asked to hear "Angel from Montgomery" (Prine, 1971, Track 4) another time. She wrote: "Which home do I go? Angleland? Pasta? The past? Angle who is?"

Harika used language like Legos pieces by color, by shape, placing words proximally together, letting them touch or crash. She gathered pieces of songs into larger meanings, sending hieroglyphic messages as defenses to be decoded (i.e., Angleland? Pasta?). We continued to revisit the concept of angels, as both a tenuous link and an attempt at obfuscation.

Harika arrived at the third session wearing a scarf her physician permitted. I offered Harika a Qur'an. She was too disappointed and irritated that it was in English to read from it. Instead, we listened to Strauss' "Sonata for Piano in B minor, Op. 5" (Strauss, 1881, Track 3). Harika's requests had become more tangible and definite (as the request for the Qur'an had been). She asked to be served soup and water in a place where diseases could be cured; then she asked me to explain the state court system. The music created a scaffold. Harika's intense affects could be held and soothed within the pieces of music, and from there we could build a common language.

She said, "I can't concentrate. These hospital people are chaos. I am alone and they don't help." She asked to be discharged to heal at her beloved temple; she referred to it as a family tradition. Harika explained that a woman from the temple had called her the day before to say the hospital was not a good place (staff reported that she had received no phone calls). "I sometimes see things in dreams," she said. "But I don't see invisible people." She continued: "If I could be in this other place, I would be better. It's the energy that heals me. Is energy the right word?" She showed, using geometrical figures, how she had gone to the temple previously seeking solitude. Harika's fantasy seemed to involve rescue by an angel who would deliver her to a place of spiritual healing, distant from suffering. Her opposite paranoid fantasy was connected to living within an intolerant host family environment, and her subsequent annihilation by abandonment in a terrifying place (Bion, 1967/1984b).

Harika and I listened to Glenn Gould playing Mendelssohn's (1834, Track 4) "Song Without Words No. 9 in E Major." She wanted to talk about the soul within the body and the layers in a person. I wondered about the conception of a psychotic break as a secular or spiritual urge to reintegrate into a new sense of self within the context of Bion's alpha function. The early infant-mother relationship involves a mother assisting an infant in establishing building blocks so growth can flourish while the infant undergoes constant integration of new experiences. This process is possible but more complex with adults who experience fragmentation and psychosis.

While we listened to Gould's "The Goldberg Variations" (Bach, 1741, Tracks 1–8) at our fourth session, Harika said, "I am very private. I don't talk to my brother or my father. She never mentioned a mother. You know more than all but two best friends in my life know about me."

Harika chose Brahms (1859, Track 13). "Intermezzo No. 2 in B-Flat Minor." She stopped the music to express her emphatic wish to leave the hospital. Harika drew a body with spots in the lungs to illustrate how water and bread could help treat diseases such as cancer. Initially, hospital staff considered Harika's request to visit a temple evidence of her delusional state. In truth, her temple was an actual place wherein she had previously found respite. Harika was trying to make sense of the dialectics—an old world and a new one, two disparate cultures, secular and spiritual, aggression and gentleness—all integrating within her. In an object relations framework, she was moving from the schizoid to the depressive position (Klein, 1946/1986).

In retrospect, Harika's resistant response to the hospital environment and her attraction to music as a form of treatment reflected historic Middle Eastern mental health treatments. Turkey has undergone dramatic modernization efforts, especially following the dissolution of the Ottoman Empire and the foundation of the modern Turkish Republic in 1923. In the Ottoman era, the health focus was on religion, not science. The predominant healers were hodjas, or teachers, found in mosques or Qur'anic schools, versed in Qur'an scriptures (Sachs, 1983; Narter, 2006). Ottoman treatment centers built in city centers were a combination of mosque, cultural school, and hospital. People who experienced madness weren't banished from community: a psychotic episode might have pointed to a quality of psyche that needed healing. Music, particularly classical Turkish music, and flowers were essential to a treatment regimen (Narter, 2006).

In modern times, Turkish women still seek non-medical treatment for mental health issues (Ozturk & Volkan, 1971; Sunter, Guz, & Peksen, 2006); these treatments adhere to ancient beliefs. Treatments often begin with prayers and consultations with a hodja. Treatments may include (Sunter, Guz, & Peksen, 2006) joining religious orders, wearing amulets, or using verses or pages from the Qur'an (p. 397). Harika's preference to visit a rural mosque was culturally appropriate. I found evidence of temples like the one Harika described, where water, bread, and soup were prescribed for typhoid, dysentery tuberculosis, and cancer. Clinicians are challenged to sit in the space of cultural differences to allow the root and nature of a patient's suffering to emerge. Harika's psychosis seemed to be a psychological dismemberment, a coming undone in the service of a self-reconstruction. I regret that I did not find at least an audio Arabic version of the Qur'an or traditional Turkish music for Harika. I could have better understood the music of her interior life.

I would have also experienced more intimately what she struggled with, in hearing and metabolizing effects of a song in a non-native language.

At the fifth session, Harika chose Beethoven's (1819–1823, Track 1) "Missa Solemnis in D Major." She covered her ears to communicate that the music was "too heavy." In the sixth session, Harika chose Gould (2003) playing Bach's (1713–1714, Track 1) "Concerto for Solo Keyboard No. 3 in D Minor (after Alessandro Marcello)." She professed to be haunted by demon voices she could not banish from her room. Harika claimed the voices disappeared when we listened to music or sat quietly. She acknowledged that music was an essential component of establishing our rapport.

I suggested that attending to sleeping and eating would enhance Harika's rehabilitation. She responded: "They, the workers here, do not want if I eat something that I really like such as desserts." She did not recall that she had initially requested a strict halal diet, which disallows animal by-products (such as cheese made from animal enzymes). Harika was only aware that she was being denied bread. She wrote:

> How can I end the invisible side? /I'm taking medicine/Stronger, less stress, trust, know future, medicine/Good friends help me, forgiveness/Qur'an would help me but they don't provide. / Brown is the stronger character/Blue is weakness and soft character/Inside blue, and outside brown. If I have my blue on the outside it will hurt me/Do I have to try to be stronger or soft?/What I have to eat?/If I have an omelet do I have to eat also bread/Or what? Or how do I have to choose my breakfast?

Harika seemed to be talking about the lack of nourishment she felt in the hospital. We did not give her the food she needed most—the Qur'an in Arabic. She pointed to a space between her eyebrows. She called it "the visionary part"; she claimed it helped distinguish inside from outside. Her sentences became less fragmented and more coherent as her inquiry shifted to explorations of vulnerability versus strength, chaos versus order, dependence versus independence, and spiritual versus medical healing.

Gradually, we were building a foundation within which to address loss and grief. Harika asked whether she could eat lunch while we listened to *The Best of Leonard Cohen* (1975, Various Tracks). After listening to a few songs she said, "A little the same. He is always sad." Next she chose Sinatra's "My Way" (Anka, Francoise, & Revaux, 1967, Track 20), and Dusty Springfield's "Son of a Preacher Man" (Hurley & Wilkinson, 1968, Track 3). She preferred lighter songs, easier to process, which made me wonder whether unsettling emotions were emerging as her psychosis diminished.

We talked about trust. Harika did not trust her host family except for the host family's daughter. She craved feeling safe. She selected the Introit of

Mozart's "Requiem" (1791, Track 1), then shut it off. "It is all death," she said. I asked if she experienced feelings that matched the music. We had been walking around the topic of grief, dipping into pavannes and requiems since we had started the music sessions.

Harika told this story in response. Seven years prior to her hospitalization, her best friend, Basimah, whom she had met at a spiritual retreat, was killed by a rejected suitor days before her scheduled wedding day. Harika recalled her shock, hearing of Basimah's death. Harika described Basimah as "young and idealistic." Harika's family had forbidden Harika from attending the funeral or visiting Basimah's grave. Harika had a fever at the time of the funeral. She admitted her grief had been frozen, unprocessed. "See, I am shaking now," she said.

We sat quietly. Harika said, "Maybe my purpose is to return home and find a husband to marry, like Basimah." I heard her fantasy of stepping into her friend's unfulfilled dream, uniting with her, and saving her friend and herself from annihilation. Harika cried and pushed her lunch away. "Why is it important? How would it be helpful to me or others?" We talked about the metaphor of unresolved grief as a dam on a river.

Later that day, a staff member requested I return to meet with Harika again. I found her kneeling on a towel by the back door. She was weeping. She said, "I want to go outside." Once there, Harika admitted feeling upset about the death of Basimah. She cried, staring off at the fence that surrounded the courtyard. Harika asked me to select music. I chose Gould (2003) performing Mendelssohn's (1830, Track 5) "Song Without Words 19b in E Major." Harika cried while the music played. It began to rain lightly; birds were singing. The bird songs seemed to move in rhythmic relationship to the Mendelssohn music. Harika asked if the birds singing were real. I told her I could also hear the birds. We talked about Basimah, and then listened quietly to a Mendelssohn piece on *Glenn Gould and Serenity* (2003). This marked a turning point in the treatment. Music critic Ralph Hill (1931) observed in *Gramophone* eighty years ago that Mendelssohn saw music as being less "ambiguous, vague and unintelligible than language" (Hill, 1931 online). He hoped people could experience connected meanings that would awaken spontaneously, without prompting by words.

Harika was upset at the start of the ninth session, which followed an occupational therapy class in which patients picked a preferred animal and tree. She said, "I misrepresented myself, I feel like an eagle even though I said seagull. My heart is more like a blueberry." She associated blueberries with peace, or as symbols for the heart. Harika explained that the black students in her college classes pushed her to be aggressive and to show eagle strength. "But I am a blueberry." She placed one hand over her heart. It was unclear whether she had tried to join with American Muslim students, only to discover cultural and political differences. I asked Harika if someone could possess qualities of both peace and strength. I wanted to understand how the death of Basimah was linked to her experiences at college and the interplay of violence and vulnerability in her mind. I noticed my own dread, as she spoke.

"You didn't know what I was like before I was here," Harika said. "You would have seen me as very strong and serious." She drew two circles on a piece of paper. Pointing to each one she said, "Eagle is CIA, and blueberry is FBI." She asked if I were a member of the FBI because I had a peaceful heart.

"The heart is peaceful," Harika said. "The mind is strong. There is so much pressure from the outside to be an eagle. But I have to follow my heart." She said that she had been somewhat paranoid since childhood and had confided in only two friends. Otherwise, she didn't let herself be known. Did her reticence protect her vulnerability, a secret transgression or fantasy of transgression she could not share? There were threads of exploration for ongoing clinical work.

Harika's choice of music allowed access, albeit limited, to her inner life. We often listened to Glenn Gould with whom Harika shared a preference for silence over the day-to-day small talk and clatter of the world. Gould embodied a great sensitivity and technical ability. He cherished a sentimental past (such as a beloved chair, handmade by his father) while also experimenting with recording technology (Ostwald, 1997). Harika liked the "Goldberg Variations" (Bach, 1741), which seemed like the verbal variations and repetitions Harika first used when bringing fragments into an integrated whole. I sensed that Harika's mind wanted to find a transcendent aesthetic form but was split between an ancient, traditional world touched by trauma and grief, and a modern world in which she experienced herself as "an other."

Harika was more able to articulate emotions in a structured fashion by the final session. She arrived at the last meeting carrying an Arabic version of the Qur'an with a red cover and gold embossed lettering. She had borrowed the book from a Muslim friend from college. The friend had also provided pink wireless earphones and an MP3 player filled with Qur'an recordings. Harika said that she found the recordings "too factual." She preferred the red book. "What my soul needs is something sweet," she said.

The Qur'an, Harika explained, inspired her to feel calm and closer to God who accepted her faults. Harika chose Sarah Brightman singing "Ave Maria" (Bach & Gounod, 1859, Track 1). She scowled then changed to baroque music. "I don't want such high voices now," she explained. She next selected Vivaldi's (circa 1741, Track 8) "Cum Dederit Delectis Suis Somnum" and then switched to Handel's (1739, Track 10) "Concerto Grosso in A Minor." She was restless. She chose a Bach piece, and then switched back to Vivaldi. Nothing was working.

Harika silenced the music and read aloud from the Qur'an. There was a steady, sonorous quality to her voice similar to the pieces of classical music she preferred. Even with more ego structure, Harika was quite interested in what was infinite and indefinable. She looked up periodically to see if I was following along. I listened intently for sounds and words that signified comfort and serenity for her.

When we began the exit Rorschach assessment, Harika became reserved again. The inkblots threatened the trust we had established. Her answers, much like in her initial test, were focused on angels. After we had completed the protocol, I asked Harika about her impressions. She said, "I feel angry at you but I am not sure why. When you asked me about the cards, I had anger rise up." This was the most directly she had expressed present tense feelings. I assured Harika that the test would not delay her hospital discharge. She asked about the court system. As we discussed her involuntary hospitalization, Harika said that she saw no difference between "spiritual seeing" and "psychosis." Harika experienced herself as being closer to God or an Absolute Truth. Eigen (1993) in "The Psychotic Core" noted that hallucinatory events might turn out to be "a gateway to the transforming power of numinosum" (p. 55). Harika wanted to make meaning from her experience.

I asked Harika if she saw exclusively angels. She admitted that she saw other figures—saying "angel" was safer. One card seemed more ominous, monstrous. We reviewed the cards: on the second pass her responses varied. She saw more animals.

Harika observed that listening to music and talking calmed her when she felt disoriented in the hospital. "Being in this place makes me want to study psychology again," she said. "Maybe that's a reason I'm here." She had studied psychology during her first attempt at college prior to her friend's death. She had been asking Allah for clarity. "These days in my country people are not given therapy in traditional ways. They are locked up," she said. She wondered who could teach her about the "unconscious."

Like many of the patients who come to the hospital on involuntary holds, Harika was caught in an acute crisis. It was initially hard to differentiate whether it was reactive or chronic. Haasen, Yagdiran, Schwartz, and Krausz (2000) remarked that a psychosis reaction to stress may be more characteristic in some non-western cultures (p. 125). In her post-Rorschach test, Harika showed up as having a PTSD/HIV constellation with high vigilance. This result could have been stimulated by past traumatic experiences, by cultural and psychological isolation and challenges with her host family. Harika was a young woman with delicate sensibilities who seemed caught in the same split as her culture. She had one foot in ancient practices, and one foot in a world of fast-paced globalization. She was also split between orthodox restraint and modern desire, passion, and shame, violence and vulnerability, and between past grief and present guilt.

Harika wanted to avoid anti-psychotic medications (although she took them each day) and involuntary detainment: she craved softer methods of rebalancing. Music seemed to fit her aesthetics. While I was reflecting on her case, I was drawn to the philosophy of fifteenth-century Italian poet Marsilio Ficino (as cited in Boer's 1980 translation), who considered music as resembling the spirit and as an essential element for healing the spirit. When Harika addressed feelings of isolation and unresolved mourning for the shocking death of her friend Basimah, it was music that stimulated grief and provided solace from the pain of grief. Harika was also helped by the containment music offered in mediating interpersonal connections formed by unconscious associations.

As we noted in an earlier chapter, Bion (1950/1984e; 1984i) observed that psychosis is forged by an early development in which there is too much tension, frustration, and arousal, with too little nurturing containment by a caring reflective internal and external environment. Seen through another lens (Jung, 1956/1977), psychosis could be considered part of the individuation process, wherein an individual can reorganize through a regressive unconscious recycling process into a new personal manifestation. Bosnak (2007), a Jungian scholar, linked this reorganization of self to complexity theory to show how a creative process might emerge from being on the verge of losing control. In complexity theory, ecosystems being both "cohesive and complex" have a tendency to "self-organize" into more complex patterns (Bosnak, 2007, p. 15).

In Bion's later years (1965), he came to believe that a regression, or disorganization through primary process thinking, could lead to transformation. Without stating it as directly as Jung or Bosnak, he considered the inscrutable aspects of human consciousness, and the limits of our knowledge. He wanted to expand the framework within which we describe potential human experience. Where I could not connect with Harika using words, music allowed a portal—for therapeutic rapport—to open. Harika trusted music when language could not make and carry meaning. Bion (1965) perceived that communication with patients in psychosis might be more like "musical or artistic" as opposed to verbal (p. 41). We built song by song, session by session, toward sitting together in grief. Music had provided a structure within which Harika could match a feeling and a thought, without threat from demon fears. She could address the deep, abiding, and fracturing grief from the loss of Basimah.

Chapter 5

Imaginary Nightclub as Potential Space

Anna stood up to dance. She gestured toward a corner surveillance camera, saying "I see you there. I know you're telling her I'm a bitch. Come over here and say it," She addressed walls as if they were windows to people from her past: "I know you're watching me in here. I'm not yours now." The room seemed transformed into a nightclub. When the song finished, she picked up the iPod to choose the next song.

"J-Lo" she sang-spoke the name. She listened to a song. "Is that all you got?" Anna said, "That's better" when she found "Walking on Sunshine" (Lopez, Winans, Combs et al., 2002, Track 1). She returned to dancing, pantomiming a striptease on a pole. The dance felt alternately seductive, competitive, and controlling. Anna was the DJ, the choreographer, and the scientist. I had the sensation of being on trial, or being tested.

In this chapter I will explore ways in which musical therapeutic space can parallel the concept of potential space (Winnicott, 1968, 1971). A therapist can build rapport with a patient by paying attention to and tending this creative space. Anna established the play space between fantasy and reality as a nightclub in which she would also later locate dimensions of her trauma. This space inherently mirrored a mother-infant space in which Anna was both mother and child.

Hug and Lohne (2009) gave the name "Third Area" to their own version of a creative working space. They postulated that having an auxiliary object (a second clinician) in the room could help create a bond by avoiding intense, direct focus on a patient. A personal listening device, such as an iPod, could serve as another auxiliary object with the added benefit of being an already trusted and familiar object for patients.

Engagement is important and difficult with people experiencing severe mental health issues (Wright, Turkington, Kingdon, & Basco, 2009).

Music can soften this difficult task. Listening to self-selected music with patients can help scaffold potential space on two levels. First, the music expresses a level of already articulated emotion the therapist is receiving as witness observer. Secondly, the clinician can more calmly attend to what is being transferred through the patient's response to the music, while the therapist can simultaneously be aware of her own "embodied countertransferences" (Samuels, 1985) to the music, the patient, and the patient's responses.

Samuels (1985) referred to embodied countertransference as the "physical, actual, material, sensual expression in the analyst of something in the patient's inner world." Possible therapist responses are falling asleep, feeling anger, or having fantasy responses such as the sensory rich image of a bird in flight. Stone (2006) offered a more musical metaphor for how therapists could pay attention to their own bodily responses: he used the image of a therapist acting as a "tuning fork" to a patient's unconscious material. Attending to embodied countertransference is especially helpful with patients, like Anna, who have suffered preverbal trauma, which haven't yet been translated to language (McDougall, 1978).

Through Anna's story, we can see the impact of early trauma on the emergence and development of psychosis. Researchers have proposed that "societal as well as familial dysfunction, abuse and trauma" may be important precursors of a psychotic disorder (Read, Mosher, & Bentall, 2004; Wittman & Keshavan, 2007). Furthermore, psychiatric hospitalization may exacerbate a patient's PTSD in an effort to address and ameliorate a crisis situation. (Wright, Turkington, Kingdon, Basco, 2009).

Anna's dances seemed to portray the kinds of traumatic experiences that psychosis might defend against rising into consciousness. Anna initially showed up naked at a Portland, Oregon, ER, after her release from jail. She was disorganized and hyper-religious. She heard voices. She had stopped taking Lithobid, Risperdal, and trazodone.

Anna, who claimed she was "half–Hong Kong" and "half Tijuana," had been living on the streets. Her first suicide attempt had occurred as a teenager in response to Tupac Shakur's death. Recently she had overdosed on Seroquel. Her sister, who managed Anna's disability checks, had involuntarily admitted Anna to the hospital claiming Anna hit her. Anna's version of the story: "I was trying to climb my family tree." Anna mentioned worries about her daughter who lived with Anna's family.

Anna's own childhood had been full of abuse by her father and others. "I was raped and beat up as a kid. No one reported it. I think I'm a little bit weirdo because of it," she told me the first time we talked. Anna dropped out of school at fifteen. Two years was the longest she had ever held a job, as well as her longest time without substances.

Lacanian scholars Davoine and Gaudillière (2004) proposed that a retreat into madness might be a normal choice for survival for someone like Anna, caught in a wheel of intense, ongoing trauma in an untenable environment. Davoine and Gaudillière (2004) refer to a "normal craziness" that "bears witness to a normality that is crazy, trivialized, de-historicized and denied." Even a place to locate the trauma "vanishes with the past: there is no place, no past, it has become impossible to trust one's own emotions and sensations" (Davoine & Gaudillière, 2004, p. 48).

That said, there are particular challenges of engagement that people experiencing psychosis face when sitting with a clinician. Participating in therapy asks a patient to tolerate sitting with her darkest, most painful feelings. Likewise, therapists are equally challenged to contain projections being pushed at them by patients experiencing psychosis—emotional states such as horror, despair, emptiness, aggression, deadness, or lack of contact with an emotional inner life. Therapists are challenged to stay anchored with the patient, while simultaneously experiencing the patients' feelings and their own countertransference feelings of overwhelming dread or disorganization.

Tustin (1972) offered sage advice on embracing a psychiatric patient's physical responses. She wrote, "The interpretation of primitive bodily states requires the capacity to enter into someone else's physical states without losing one's head." What Tustin calls "interpretation" here seems more aptly described by Bion (1990), and later theorists (Grotstein, 2007; Charles, 2012) using the metaphor of bringing "a penetrating beam of darkness" into the primitive parts of the mind and preverbal emotional states of the patient. As I have previously noted, music can help create and maintain a safe space of reverie wherein a therapist can remain calm and centered while helping a patient to digest distressing emotions through words, symbols or actions. This can be tedious, exhausting work in the company of another: to sit with deafening emptiness, within an unbridgeable void. At the same time, it is a respectful, humane gesture: one that is likely of value to all parties involved.

An attuned clinician has an opportunity to help patients make use of their music more conscious and deliberate. Reich (1972, 1973), among others (McDougall, 1978), posited that the unconscious was communicated in physical gestures, postures, facial expressions, and somatic symptoms. Per Reich, presence and attentiveness allowed a clinician to note the transference, or the unconscious, archaic images the patient imposed on the therapist. Likewise, a therapist could more easily discern countertransference in her own unconscious reactions to patients, in addition to her own ideation and transference. With Anna, I felt uncertainty, and vigilance.

Anna's presentation was bizarre and unpredictable throughout her hospitalization. She used felt-tip markers for makeup. She took showers clothed. She walked into other patients' rooms to borrow clothes. When told to wait for a smoke break she said: "You guys are all going to get murdered when I get out of here." Then, she laughed, to undercut her threat. Anna's family members preferred she live in a state hospital. It is not surprising she mistrusted them. She worried that her sister was stealing her identification card or money. She called 911 twice.

"I think I'm schizo," Anna told staff. Frightened of her hallucinations, Anna requested to share her room rather than be alone. She seldom used language to express pain. She seemed to process emotions through somatic symptoms, often complaining of stomach cramps, ankle and neck pain, and general agitation.

When I approached her about music, she asked. "How much do I get paid? Does it get me extra cigarettes?" I explained the purpose and possible benefits of the study. She said, "Is this my film contract? Camera please." I went over the contract with her, while she played with her hair. "Blah, blah, blah," she said, "Why don't you just show me where to sign." I gave her the contract to read overnight.

The next day she had thrown the contract away. We finished a second version. Anna called the Rorscharch "A big mess, but maybe it will make sense to you if you wear 3-D glasses." I asked her to list music that she wanted downloaded. "Oh yeah," she said, "Start writing these down." She first suggested R & B and rap artists—J-Lo, Shakira, Missy Elliot, Jim Jones, DMX, Poison—and Billy Joel. She reviewed the list: "OK thanks, Lindsay. Get me that and an MP3 player." I reminded her my name is Trisha.

Anna, like most patients experiencing psychosis I encountered, had an already-established strong rapport with music. Patients often use music instinctively for such purposes as self-expression, emotional modulation, diversion, and emotional containment. Music can circumvent cognitive defenses and distortions and communicate directly with the body (Rose, 2004). A therapist using music as an adjunct tool can gain insight into a patient by being present for the physical conversation that takes place through incremental shifts and tangible gestures.

Anna used gestures and behaviors to show movement between various self-states—from ironic clarity, to delusional, to playful, to bizarre, and sometimes disorganized—during her nightclub performances. From the very first session she always faced the surveillance cameras. This gesture seemed to symbolize her attitude toward the cold eyes she perceived judging her: in her family, in the social framework in which she was pinned, and in the research sessions. Anna always seemed to be asking me whether I was part of her internalized critic or an ally?

Anna performed, and then sat down. After a long pause, she asked, "Are we going to talk now or what?" She told me it was her friend's birthday. "I miss her so much. You look a little like her. She was loyal. That's why

I trusted you." Then Anna stood abruptly and asked for an Usher song. I had "Love in This Club" (Usher et al., 2008, Track 1). She grimaced, "That's a hard one. It reminds me of a super-ass who cheated on me with my little sister. I should have hit her. Joke. She wanted to be me. So I stole her ID."

Anna listened to half the song, then sat down again. "I'll tell you about my grandpa. He was really good. He spoiled my sister and me when we were little. When he died," Anna continued, "everything changed, it was much harder. My father wasn't supportive. He wears cowboy boots like yours. Are those his boots?"

Anna said she was done talking. She selected Michael Jackson's *(1983, Track 5)* "Beat It," singing in call-and-response, "Egg, egg, egg," each time the refrain came around. She laughed at her own joke, then tired of it and switched to a Justin Timberlake song. She sat down to listen, closing her eyes, folding her hands across her belly. "I liked this song much better when I was fucked up," she said. The song was not the escape she longed for. It did not comfort. It would not conjure up a lost pleasurable moment.

For Anna and many people with psychosis, no early mechanism was established for breaking down experience into digestible pieces (Bion, 1967/1984). There were no words or other symbolic containers to express experiences. Without sufficient caregiver mediation in breaking down sensations, and emotions, and digesting them through the help of a caregiver's imagination, fantasy, illusion, and symbolization, an infant may become overwhelmed beyond her nervous system threshold capacity (McEwen, 2003; Mulvihill, 2005; Nijenhuis, 2004). Considering also that people who experience psychosis are highly sensitive to environmental stimuli, early developmental or environmental trauma may have led them to pathological states (Bion, 1984; Schore, 1994, 2002, van der Kolk, Roth, Pelcovitz, Sunday, & Spinazzola, 2005).

Anna, like other patients who struggle with psychosis, seemed to defend against unbearable feelings through increased primary process thinking (Freud, 1957) not subject to the rules of logic or oriented to reality (i.e., dreams, hallucinations). She also seemed to experience increased intrusion of implicit, unconscious memories, and increased intense unbounded emotions, which have been associated with increased right hemisphereic activity (Cozolino, 2002). Anna struggled with a strong sense of isolation and lack of ability to join safely with others (Rosenbaum, 2005). She had alienated her family, including her own daughter, and had trouble connecting to people.

When I fetched Anna for the second session, she was lying tangled in bed sheets on the thin mattress she had pulled off its wooden platform. She greeted me as Lindsay. I reminded her again that my name is Trisha. She replied, "Okay Lindsay, whatever you want to call yourself today." She covered one nostril and took a quick snort. Then she winked. "Just bring your little stereo in here," she said. I suggested we go to a meeting room. I waited. She emerged minutes later, wearing her bedspread as a cape. Once we were settled in a room, she picked a song and then said, "Just pretend I'm dancing."

For the third session, I found Anna in the dayroom wearing a tight red sweatshirt. Her roommate was yelling about a stolen sweatshirt. Anna, oblivious, focused intently on watching Lady Gaga on TV. "She's ugly," Anna said, "Like some dog chewed Madonna up and they just glued her back together." Someone laughed. Anna said, "See . . . you know what I mean." Her phrasing was always syncopated, rhythmic, musical and inviting with a quick disconnect, or drop, at the end.

"Hi Lindsay," she said, when she saw me. "You pick some stuff this time," she said, "But if it sucks I'll push you aside. No, no cowboy shit," she said after a few bars of a Johnny Cash song, "You can listen to that with my father, I can't dance to that shit."

I switched to Beyoncé and Shakira singing, "Beautiful Liar" (Eriksen, Hermandsen, Ghost, Dench, & Knowles, 2007). "That's more like it," Anna said. She stood up shaking her hair back and forth. "I know you're looking at me," she said to the security camera and to those of us who locked her up literally and metaphorically. "It's no secret. I know you talk behind my back and start rumors. You think I give a shit?" She turned her back on the camera and marched across the room to look through a small window in the door. "I'm in the middle here," she said, "You're outside. He's behind glass. I'll do what I want." She shimmied between the security camera and the door.

Anna seemed to be performing her trauma—and her subsequent disappearance into a fantasy, a nightclub world where she escaped in her mind, and where she had concretely escaped in the past, with the help of substances. Did she envision her father? Was I her father, or her sister stealing her identity? Was I a perpetrator, an exploiter or a friend? She was asking about trust. I felt pinned to my chair: on alert, on edge, not knowing what might happen next—a feeling with which I was certain Anna was intimate.

"Okay, Lindsay," she said, " I'm done with that song. Give me a new one." I picked Jackson's (Porcaro & Bettis, 1983, Track 7) "Human Nature." She traced delicate hand gestures as if holding small flags. She sang: "Why, why, de da da da de da da da," marching back and forth, and waving to an imaginary audience. Something about that song choice allowed Anna to release the utilitarian exchange of the nightclub and enter a different self-state of innocence and play. I wondered if she felt safer?

When I approached her for the fourth session, she asked, "Did you bring me a soda?" It was 9:00 AM. Anna paced the hallway with a towel wrapped around her head, waiting for her morning medication. "I need something slow this morning," she said when we sat down. "Why don't you pick out something Lindsay?" I chose Bob Marley, "One Love" (Marley & Mayfield, 1984, Track 8).

"Nice work," she said. She swayed back and forth singing loudly, "Let's get together and be alright." She asked me to join in singing. Then she chose Lil Wayne's "Drop the World" (Carter, 2009, Track 8). She paced in front of the camera. "That song makes you feel," she said. She chanted along, rapping Portland area codes.

"Why haven't my friends come to visit me?" she asked later. "Even my daughter didn't come. Where's my father? He just got out but he's back." She changed the song's chorus to letting the world crash on someone's (maybe my?) "fucking head." Anna seemed angry at her abandoning family and at my lack of helpfulness in motivating her family to visit. The song finished. She scrolled through the iPod again, selecting Jackson's "Bad" (Jackson, 1987, Track 1). She started her dance with eyes closed, arms by her sides. "This one is positive energy for followers," she said. "It's not negative like people might think." She made a paradoxical gesture of shooting a gun.

When sitting with Anna, I sensed that we were co-creating a third area. The iPod was one object, the surveillance camera—another one; both objects set the perimeters of our creative space. Gesture and language were part of the musical navigation between us: a call and response. The past and the present, ancestors, family, and friends all merged in the room (Davoine & Gaudillière, 2004). Anna allowed me to bear witness to layers of trauma, violence, and destructive influences that made her internal and external worlds dangerous. She affirmed the need for caution because of destructive memories that returned: men with guns, voices and intrusive visions.

Davoine and Gaudillière (2004) explained the transmission of traumas by noting that when experiencing trauma a patient is not "limited to his brain case and the neurons it encloses"; they suggested taking into account "ancestors and living relatives, with whom a patient was related by means of various language games" (p. 51). Sometimes they noticed, as did McDougall (1989), that trauma was transmitted by the absence of words, emotions, and the absence of language itself.

"Pick a last one," Anna said, "Something soft like the way we started." I chose Al Green singing "Belle" (Green, Jordan, & Fairfax, Jr., 1977, Track 1). When the song finished she asked: "This one makes you happy again?" She was inquiring if the song, like the sessions, were for my behalf or hers? Did we have any basis for trust?

Music may be better suited than language to address unbounded implicit memories or other psychotic defenses while a therapist is learning to attune to a patient's rhythm. It is possible that psychosis may be, among other things, an unconscious method, a strategy with which to face unbearable losses (Lewis, 2004). Selecting a particular song could help express a brief release or regulation of a dreaded emotion such as grief or rage. One example of this might be Anna's choice of Lil Wayne's "Drop the World" (Carter, 2009) in which that singer fantasizes about annihilation.

Anna sang en route to her sixth session. "Don't be glaring at me," she said to another patient. "I ain't the devil. Hey Lindsay," she turned toward me. "Did you bring a soda?" I told her I brought music. "I'd rather have soda," she said. I asked why she called me Lindsay. "Don't ask, Redhead, you know. Going to the clubs . . ." She snorted. I finally realized she meant Lindsay Lohan. This opened the concept of a twinship dimension to our interactions (Kohut, 1972). In sharing her clubbing experiences, Anna had linked me to Lohan, who, like Anna, acted out emotions in public, under constant surveillance.

Anna asked, "When does the last Dexter come out?" She referred to a TV show about an antisocial character who performed forensic investigations and strategical murders. I wondered if she linked the character to my metaphorically dismembering analysis. I told her the show had ended. "Well shit, I missed it," she said. She was irritable. She chose "Beautiful Liar" (Eriksen et al., 2007), but soon marched over to the iPod to stop it. "I'm sick of that church," she said. She chose DMX, singing "Lord Show Me A Sign" *(Simmon & Storch, 2006, Track 1).* "That's more my speed," Anna said, "Harder." She asserted control over the space. Then she sat down beside me, suddenly focused and clear. "Do you want to hear about my life or what?" she asked. "I was born in 1976 in Vancouver. My mom was abusive. My father beat us up. I had a bunch of cousins, aunts and uncles who spoiled me. She said, "Get it right Lindsay. You're only gonna have this chance." She continued, "Lala was my favorite cousin. She's in heaven because her stomach exploded at thirty and she had no money to fix it. My sister has social security and food stamps." She repeated louder, "Food stamps." She stood up to pace. "I wanted to take my daughter. I called and she said, 'Not for a week Mamma', but I say Monday." She interrupted herself: "Hey it's Sunday tomorrow. We should go to church." Her visiting defense lawyer interrupted the session. "Let's meet again later," she said, "I need to talk . . . bring a soda, K? Sprite." A nurse remarked that Anna had stopped taking showers while fully clothed.

Anna yelled from the nurses' station, "Hey Lindsay. Don't stand me up." I asked her why she slept on the floor. She explained that three wooden boxes, side by side, reminded her of a graveyard: "It's better to sleep on the floor than be in the grave." She put on DMX's "Lord Show Me A Sign" (*Simmon & Storch, 2006, Track 1).* "This is the real radio," she said, "It's the energy. A place I know. You know it, Lindsay." The reference was ambivalent but clear. We shared a project. We could go to church, and build rapport. We witnessed trauma in the room, in the music, and in her history. Anna didn't stay on one subject. She was manic. "Your boots," she said, "My dad says, I like me a cowgirl." The link to her father indicated that I was dangerous again. I felt wary, wondering what she planned.

During a Tupac Shakur song Anna said her voices were speaking through me. She suggested I hold them while she danced. Was I also holding her self-destructive urges, rage, and grief? She seemed lost. She watched the camera while touching the walls, as if trying to locate something in the environment that she felt internally. She rubbed her hands over her belly. "You know I could be pregnant," she said, "Maybe I need a test."

"You have a new life inside of you?" I asked. The question intruded on the space as if I were trying to, steal her creativity or know too much—more than her meaning (Winnicott, 1971)

Anna stared at me with her head cocked to the side. She shook her head; I had missed her message. "My family hasn't come. I think I need some J-Lo or Lloyd. Pick me out something nice?" she said, then, "You remind me of my friend, Jody."

"Was that a hard meeting with your lawyer?" I asked

"He just talked and had me sign things," she said, "Just like you, Lindsay. He said ninety days, blah, blah, . . . state hospital blah . . . your daughter, blah, blah. I smashed a can after he left," she said, "But there was still coke in it, so uh oh." She made the sign of the cross then whispered, "Tell the security camera to quit talking behind her back." She was allowing them all in the room: family, voices, memories, images, and affects.

"Pick a song for my second husband," she said. I picked OMC, "How Bizarre" (Jansson & Fuemana, 1995, Track 1). Anna said, "That's REAL old school." She stood up with her head high like a club proprietor. She strutted around the room, looked through the door window, and said, "We're all full. Go down the street or come back later." Pretending the iPod was her phone, she waved me away: "I have a date. We'll talk later."

Listening to preferred music with a therapist may help patients, like Anna, develop a safe container in a relational setting precisely because music has a particularly relaxing and organizing effect (Glickson & Cohen, 2000; Neilzen & Cesarec, 1981). Music may also better diminish negative symptoms such as depression and anxiety, than can more behavioral interventions (Gold, Solli, Krüger, & Lie, 2009; Mössler, Chen, Heldal, & Gold, 2011). Music can also better build a common ground for interpersonal connections, such as Anna's created nightclub space in which she and I could meet (Ulrich, Houtmans & Gold, 2007).

At the eighth session, Anna asked to meet in her room. She was lying on her mattress. "I keep crying," she said. "My family hasn't come. How long have I been here Lindsay?" I told her a month. She buried her face in her pillow, crying again. Then she selected a UB40 song. "It reminds me of my first husband, Paco," she said. "He sang to me. Sometimes he hit me. Only when he was high." She asked for a change. I selected Iz singing "What A Wonderful World" (Thiele & Weiss, 1967, Track 2). "Kind of cheesy, Lindsay," she said, "But nice lullaby voice." She asked for more Iz, and then fell asleep.

Anna paced the halls before the ninth session. She wore pink flip-flops; her hair was tied back in a bun. She asked to borrow reading glasses. I had an extra pair. She chose Lloyd's "Get It Shawty" (Lackey et al., 2007) danced a few bars, then sat down.

"I wanna talk to you," she said, "Where's the money? Just kidding." She laughed, "Did you bring me a soda?" I commented about her need for exchange.

"That's the way it is Lindsay," she said, "You give ta get, get ta give . . . give it. She kissed a rough patch of caulked paint on the wall. She accepted imaginary money, put it in her bra, and then took it out. "Where's my commission?" she asked. Anna puffed up her chest, and threw back her shoulders as she walked toward the security camera. She asked, "Did my father bring me cigarettes? Her pants were on backward with plastic zip ties through belt loops. She held up her pants with her hand "Can you help me?" she requested, "I want to dance but they're falling down."

What came to mind when witnessing Anna's regressions in terms of her sleeping on the floor and hunting for siblings' clothes was Sullivan's (1953) concept of parataxis, wherein early childhood experiences are undergone as momentary unconnected states of being. Anna showed the abandonment she felt within her family. Her father was in prison. Her siblings were rivals. Her body had sexual value or else it was discardable.

I found zip ties and helped her fortify a makeshift belt. "Thanks, Lindsay," she said. "I hope they don't put you in the jail hospital Monday" as if we were twins who would be switching places. She told me she would leave the hospital on Monday to return to her own apartment, contrary to what was written in her chart. I handed her the iPod and reading glasses. "We have the same color hair," she said. (Mine was red, hers jet black.) "Are we from the same family?" The music seemed to wash by her. She said, "Hey let's go ask Blondie about cigarettes."

I suggested we finish the music session. She mimicked me. I scratched my left arm; she scratched hers. She pretended to hide imaginary money in her bra. "I have $100,000," she said. "I called my best friend and she's going to come here."

I have wondered, as relational theorists have suggested, whether pathologies like psychosis are more likely to be resolved in a relational field with a clinician rather than intraspychically (Stolorow & Stolorow, 1987). It is doubtful that Anna would have continued to meet if it weren't for the music aspects of the sessions. Choosing and responding to music allowed her to be more in control. She could reveal what she wanted, in the process of a game she controlled, at her own pace.

Before her last session, I learned that Anna had stopped taking medications to prepare for a court appearance. I found her dancing in the dayroom, her pants on backward again. She asked if I had remembered her soda and hamburger. She chose a song and danced facing the surveillance cameras, and the TV screen. She ran her hands across every surface. Then she peered through the door peephole and returned to the whiteboard to draw a mandala. It looked like a Star of David with an eye in the middle surrounded by two cloudlike circles. "It's energy," she said. She continued to stare at the whiteboard as the next song by UB40 played. "It's a resurrection," she said.

"Yours?" I asked.

She replied, "Yes. How long have I been in this graveyard?" She was cold: I found her a bedspread to wrap around her shoulders. She closed her eyes. When the song finished she asked, "Do you feel that energy? Not even the hospital believes I had a miscarriage three months ago. My family doesn't care. They don't come here."

I wondered if "miscarriage" was her way of talking about trauma, or catastrophic loss. She showed me a tattoo of an angel on her back. "Angelina is my daughter's name," she said. "I am always her mother. I have always come back." She confessed a premonition that her daughter was hooking. "It's what we do in our family."

I was surprised that she sat while Jackson's, "Human Nature" *(Porcaro & Bettis, 1982, Track 7)* played. "You're quiet today," I observed.

"I'm on my period," she answered, "Very emotional and clear. God is good." I noticed she was no longer wearing felt-tip make-up. She seemed somber. "Do you believe in mummies?" she asked. Maybe you're the first mummy," She laughed. "That sounded funny."

Our potential play space had turned into a place of open conversation in which we were building a basis for attachment. Were we twins? Was she allowing me to nurture her? I thanked her for talking. She opened her eyes and replied, "Oh . . . you mean for letting you in? You're thanking me for that?" She put both hands on her head. "And where's my soda. You're testing me to see how long I can go without it."

Anna expected to leave from court the next day, so she hoped I would have gifts for her. The charge nurse told me it was highly unlikely Anna would be discharged from court. "What's more likely," she added, "Is that she'll go to the state hospital." The nurse's prediction was accurate: Anna was discharged abruptly that evening to the state hospital. She had time to pack. She left a note "You owe me a soda, Lindsay Lohan."

Music is not the only adjunct modality that might prove useful in working with individuals like Anna who have experienced, and who may be re-enacting, trauma. What is unique to music is its accessibility, and its capacity to help metabolize unsettling emotional experiences. Noting subtleties of countertransference in the potential space, which shifts shapes as it develops, can help a therapist build chains of patients' musical associations "to connect together in a meaningful way" (Dieckmann, 1974, p. 73). Such mindful attention can be especially important when working with patients like Anna who have suffered preverbal and ongoing trauma, and who prefer to communicate through actions or performances rather than through language (McDougall, 1978). Music therapists Aldridge and Fachner (2006) noted that health is performed, and that discerning truth, both individually and collectively, is also performed. They describe performance as the reconciliation of internal and external realities wherein truth is brought into consciousness.

Marilynne Robinson observed in *Absence of Mind* (2010): "Each of us lives intensely within herself, continuously assimilating past and present experience to a narrative and vision that are unique in every case, yet profoundly communicable" (p. 132). Music can be an effective portal, allowing access to this narrative/visioning process.

Chapter 6

Ramble On

Raves, Social Urges, and Psychosis

This chapter will explore building musical rapport with young adults contending with early psychosis. Music and personal listening devices are intimately tied to identity with young adults; thus music is helpful when trying to piece back together an identity fragmented by psychological crisis. Early intervention programs focus on providing intensive services throughout the first three to five years of diagnosis (McGorry, Killackey, Elkins, Lambert, & Lambert, 2003). Early psychosis responds better to treatment than do later stages of the condition.

Psychosis, particularly schizophrenia, involves disturbances in verbal language (Kestenbaum, 1986; Feinsilver, 1986; Andreasen, 1979a, 1979b; Peccecia & Benedetti, 1998) and abnormalities in the processing of auditory and visual sensory stimuli (Erlenmeyer-Kimling, 1976). Young people experiencing psychosis can borrow language—through the vehicle of self-selected music—that is already contained and harmonized in an emotionally consistent frame, to express affect. Listening to preferred music has been linked to positive change in affect and it has a purgative or cathartic effect for young adults in emotional distress (Baker & Bor, 2008; Lacourse, Claes, & Villeneuve, 2001; Martin, Clarke, & Pearce, 1993; Stack, 1998).

Music served as a diversion and source of motivation for the patients detailed in this chapter. Another common, complicating feature for each patient was a history of prolonged use of recreational drugs. Using substances such as marijuana initially helped them feel less awkward, and more autonomous while they navigated diffusive and chaotic social settings. Unfortunately, extensive use of recreational drugs can exacerbate symptoms in patients vulnerable to psychosis. Khantzian (1995) noted that although drugs relieve suffering, reliance on those drugs can also amplify that suffering.

In such precarious territory, music may be a counterbalancing force. It is already an influential one. Research studies estimated that adolescents and young adults from the US and the UK listened to music between 2.5 and four hours each day (Arnett, 1995; Rideout, Foehr, & Roberts, 2010; Tarrant, North, & Hargreaves, 2000). We cannot yet fathom how walking through life listening to a soundtrack shapes young adults' emotional experiences.

Matt, Seneca, and Elliot all struggled to construct a sense of identity while contending with the internal chaos of early psychosis complicated by substance use. Each patient had difficulty navigating social relationships, individuating from parents, and launching into adulthood responsibilities. They all shared an additional difficulty—trusting treatment providers.

Early psychosis interventions are internationally labeled as psychiatric emergencies (McGorry & Yung, 2003). Strong evidence shows that emotional dysfunctionality in such forms as depression, suicidal thinking, social anxiety, and traumatic reactions develop rapidly and intensely after a first psychotic episode or during the prodromal phase (Birchwood, Iqbal, & Chadwick, 2000; Cosoff, Julian, & Cosoff, 1998; McGorry, Chanen, McCarthy, & Van Riel, 1991). Early intervention strategies address three main areas: early detection, reduced delay in treatment, and keeping up sustained intervention over several years (Reading and Birchwood, 2005). The most highly effective treatments reduce symptoms and promote recovery from psychosis, with high probability (80–90 percent) of symptomatic recovery following a first episode of psychosis (Robinson, Woerner, & Alvil, 1999; McGorry & Yung, 2003). Although first episode interventions have mainly been conducted with schizophrenic patients, these same intervention principles could be useful for other diagnoses with psychotic features, such as bipolar disorder.

The American Psychiatric Association's Practice Guideline for the Treatment of Patients with Schizophrenia (2004) and researchers (Seligman & Reichenberger, 2007) have suggested, medication management and psychosocial interventions can best address the acute psychotic phase and residual symptoms of schizophrenia. Cognitive Behavioral Therapy (CBT) has proven helpful for clients to explore and change positive symptoms of psychosis (Dickerson, 2000), including delusions and hallucinations. CBT helps "reduce bizarre and destructive behaviors and improve functioning" (Seligman & Reichenberger, 2007, p. 499). CBT has proven less effective in reducing the negative symptoms of psychosis such as blunted affect, restricted speech, and lack of motivation (Seligman & Reichenberger, 2007).

There are increasing calls for other effective approaches for people with psychosis (Bentall, 2009; Fledderus, Bohlmeijer, Smit, & Westerhof, 2010; Herrman, Saxena, & Moodie, 2005; Slade, 2009). Depth-based interventions, focused on affect and expression, are useful (Leite, 2003). Because music in particular is shown to have such positive effects (Gold, Solli, Krüger, & Lie,

2009; Mössler, Chen, Heldal, & Gold, 2011), Norway and the UK have recommended music as part of treatment guidelines (National Collaborating Centre for Mental Health, 2010; The Norwegian Directorate of Health, 2013). A solid therapeutic relationship is also essential for patients with early psychosis (Hogarty, Greenwald, Ulrich, Kornblith, DiBarry, Cooley, & Flesher, 1997).

Hospitals provide stabilization and haven for early psychosis patients; however, detainment may also cause alienation, stress, or trauma. Feelings of being an "other" may intensify, as we observed with Harika, when a person shares space with numerous disorganized patients. For a clinician, it can be a delicate matter to join with a patient who perceives his entire environment, including providers, as dangerous. Even the smallest gesture matters. Words may carry menacing or dismissive meanings if delivered too quickly or with an impatient tone of voice. Given that psychosis can be exacerbated, as we observed with Orlando, by high emotive expressiveness or extreme responses (Hooley & Campbell, 2002; Hooley & Gotlib, 2000), it is important for clinicians to remain calm and transparent. A therapist needs to attune with focused tenderness, such as during the shared moment of a song that is saying something about transcendence, or lost love, or rage.

Matt was quite traumatized by being locked up in a psychiatric hospital. He arrived via the Detox Unit after trying to cut his wrist lengthwise while drunk. He was twenty-one, single, and white with no history of previous hospitalizations. Matt became suicidal after an embarrassing event that brought his sexuality into question. He had not slept for four days. He became isolative and quiet. Matt's behaviors worsened two weeks prior to his hospitalization. The admitting physician described Matt as responding to internal stimuli and command hallucinations. Matt paused extensively between sentences, and often lost the trail of his topic. Matt's initial diagnosis was schizoaffective with cannabis dependence. He told staff he had been drinking one-fifth bottle of vodka daily for several years. He confirmed that he consistently smoked marijuana on a recreational basis. Matt had been unemployed for over two years. He lived with his parents and attended classes to certify as a robotics technician. Once he cleared from his initial psychosis, he wanted distance from the experience of losing control in public. He initially attacked all compassionate gestures.

When I first approached Matt he was notably paranoid. He had been attending therapeutic groups several times per week, but would abruptly leave the room if anyone sat too close, or focused on him too intently. I asked him if he would be interested in a music research study, noting that several other patients had participated.

"Are you trying to pressure me to be like other people?" Matt asked. He walked away angry. The next day he approached me saying, "My doctor said it was okay to talk to you." He scrolled through the/playlists on the iPod. He asked for Suzanne Vega and Portishead, noting that he preferred the familiar acapella version of Tom's Diner (Vega, 1987c, Track 1). Matt was not sure why he had been admitted to the hospital. He observed, "I have trouble talking to girls. And I have a friend who told me he's gay." Matt spoke slowly with flat affect, and steady intonations like a low-key talk radio host. He had no history of relationships. "I was seeing a really beautiful girl," he said, "but I wasn't moving fast enough. She asked if I was gay." He paused to see how I reacted, then said, "I wondered if I was gay because she really KNEW me and she asked THAT. Now, I think I'm shy. I have trouble talking to women." When "Tom's Diner" (Vega, 1987c, Track 1) ended, Matt selected Vega's (2003, Track 15) "Calypso." He liked Vega's "straightforward and easy" voice. I wondered if the music made our conversations easier. Matt told me about his experiences with women while Vega's song played in the background: "I learned how to act confident but not too confident. Not too much eye contact but don't look away too much." He stopped to change the song and said, "I know I'm paranoid, but I CAN read other meanings into what people say. If someone is talking about Susie who went off the deep end, I think they mean me. And I'm not crazy."

In trying to understand Matt, I looked for links to unconscious material through song choices. Matt's attraction to Vega, much like Hanna's, corresponded with strong intellectual defenses, and a preference for detachment. Matt wanted Vega-style protection from unpredictable emotions. Vega's music has been described as self-contained, even self-protective: her songs have been compared to "lyrical cloaks" or "mantras:" to hide inside (Holden, 2010). Vega's music has further been described as cryptic and formal, with elements of film noir (Bowman, 2011). Perhaps for Matt, Vega was an ideal twin (Winnicott, 1972), or the ideal, unattainable woman, wounded and aloof. Vega loved femme fatale actresses with cruel streaks, like Marlene Dietrich (Source). Matt revealed his own cruel streak, which surfaced in sarcastic jokes. He was cruel to himself when under stress. His voices shared this sardonic tone.

In later sessions, Matt selected Portishead's (Gibbons, 1994c, Track 1) "Mysterons" for its steady, trance-slow rhythms. The music was well modulated like Matt's voice, or the soft poetic ballads of Vega. Matt's musical choices seemed to fulfill a missing mothering, emotional regulation function, although the reasons he might prefer lulling songs were not in his conscious awareness. Nor would it have been appropriate in such a brief encounter as ten listening sessions to explore his connection with his mother in depth. A clinician who continued to work with Matt could explore how Vega's and Portishead's rhythm, tone, and volume of vocalization helped modulate emotional pain and arousal for Matt (Beebe & Stern, 1977).

Matt always kept up a steady stream of conversation. He was uncomfortable with silence, even with music in the background. Matt explained he had wanted to study engineering but felt overwhelmed by social aspects of school. He smoked marijuana to cope, and switched to a robotics program, which combined engineering and helping people. Matt selected Portishead's song, "Numb," (Gibbons, 1994c, Track 7) and asked that I listen for the melody. It seemed that he wanted me to understand how the song conveyed his numbness. When the song ended, Matt said, "I'm falling behind in the world." I understood that to mean that he was embarrassed to live in his father's house while high school friends had children and careers.

At the next sessions, Matt picked similar Vega and Portishead music. Once the songs helped construct an initial therapeutic frame, Matt talked about intimate aspects of his life. He said, "When people are uncomfortable or scared they call me 'The Eagle,' 'The Library,' or 'Face.'" Matt believed he had a dark presence. He said, "People walk out of rooms when I enter." He was worried about having an identity crisis and about being narcissistic because he was cruel to his father. "I slice him with words," Matt said. I thought about Matt slicing his own arms, to cut out or through the cruel part of him that was his father.

"Are you afraid you might destroy someone?" I asked.

"Yes and no," he said. He talked about an occupational therapy class in which he was asked to choose between a butterfly, a fish, or a cat. He obsessed about the meaning of each choice. If he chose a cat, would the therapist think he was a hunter? Matt became overwhelmed by the emergence of unconscious associations, upon which he ruminated. I wondered with him about whether the therapist was instead interested in Matt's ability to follow directions?

"I see what you're suggesting," he said. "But I don't believe it. If I chose a butterfly she might think I was gay." Matt continued to transfer inner conflicts into imagined critical reactions by staff. He seemed dissociated from his own desires and needs. With the help of preferred music and a clinician to mitigate his anxiety, could Matt explore his fears and his anger at his spartan father and emotionally absent mother?

Matt selected Vega (1987a, Track 1) singing "Luka." He listened quietly and then said, "When I start to hear voices and get overwhelmed, I go to my room and lie down." Most of Matt's voices were critical and wanted to harm him. He had learned to compartmentalize the voices, like listening to music on low volume, so it remained background noise. He could ignore lyrics (voices), but remained aware of melody and rhythm. This worked as a temporary strategy. He noted that shared exchanges of music between us helped him feel less stuck.

Matt said, "I want to talk about how I know whether perceptions are real or not." We discussed the first time I approached Matt. He worried I would administer tests to discern if he was gay. His physician assured him I would not test for sexual preference. Revisiting that one incident (which took the length of a song) was sufficient for Matt; he next chose "Weird Fishes" by Radiohead (Yorke & Greenwood, 2007a, Track 4). Matt spoke over the layered, non-linear song, explaining his sense of foreboding when he fixed his family's computers. He worried that his mental confusion caused machines to break. As part of his lingering psychosis, Matt, like many other people struggling with schizophrenia, had difficulty distinguishing boundaries as described by Rosenbaum (2005) of inside and outside, self and other, and even self and object. Music allowed him space to risk revealing the ways his mind seemed unreliable to him.

"I bring other people down," he said. He sensed that his face was repulsive and fear-inducing to others because it conveyed to the world what was inside him—darkness and voices. Matt sensed that his father wasn't afraid of him, but that he hovered, and tried to live vicariously through Matt. He attacked to keep his father at a distance. Matt's fantasies were of mythic proportions, in contrast to the ordinary world in which he was disorganized and forgetful. Could the two worlds be brought together with music as a background? Could he tolerate the anxiety? Could I help him gradually learn tolerance?

"I'm sorry," he said, as we stood up to leave. "I can't remember your name."

In the fifth session, with Portishead as background, Matt spoke about his high school rugby career. He seemed to be slowly growing to trust me; he allowed for longer periods of silence, and said he hoped that our ease in conversation would translate into future interactions with women. He wondered whether people would be easier if they were logical like machines? "People are harder to predict," he said. "You expect X and they do something that feels and looks like K." We experimented next, by surprise, with weathering disappointment.

Matt forgot about my planned absence over a weekend. He assumed that I was displeased and avoiding him. The following Tuesday, as we listened to Prodigy's "Climbatize" (Howlett, 1997, Track 9), Matt was bothered by the loud volume, equivalent to the rupture which caused dissonance in our attunement. Matt manipulated the iPod to avoid frustration. He adjusted dials mumbling, "What does this do?" I had proven more inscrutable than a machine. I told Matt I had listened to Portishead over the weekend. He replied "I don't really care what people think of me anymore." We had not resolved the abandonment issue. Matt talked about his brother—an engineer who built libraries in Africa—who was visiting along with a niece he teased about being pregnant when she was not.

"I'm sarcastic," he said, "and I have a very serious face." I reflected back to him that he was smiling. He seemed detached from his own affective responses (Bion, 1984), although he was also quite playful during sessions. Music in the background helped modulate his emotions.

"Wait," he said. He held down the sides of his mouth, and then let them go. "I can't make small talk with people around here anymore. People just talk AT me."

While we listened to Portishead, he described having a nice conversation with a nurse, but not knowing how to end it. Wanting to try something new, he said to her, "I don't know what to say now." She told him to say "Nice to talk with you." He was satisfied but later worried she was mocking him. He retreated until his anxiety lifted.

After seven sessions, we reached a place of provincial trust wherein Matt started taking musical risks. He scrolled meticulously through each artist on the iPod. He mumbled a running commentary: "Don't know. That's a maybe." He settled on Miles Davis,' "So What" (Davis, 1959, Track 1). "It's a little like trance music," he said. Davis' music had cool, detached rhythms and technically perfect improvisations.

Matt continued, "I had some bad experiences with girls, then I was angry about women, but less now." He gave an example of misunderstood sarcasm: "If I said, 'your hair looks nice today,' you could take that as a compliment but really your hair is messy so it's sarcastic."

"I get it," I replied. "But then if I don't laugh or don't show you that I get the joke, you worry about what I'm thinking."

"That's it," he said. We talked about deducing through gesture, tone of voice and facial expression, if a message arrived close to its intended meaning. For a clinician, continuing to work with Matt, it would be useful to explore how to engage in social activities in a manner less threatening to his fragile ego. Next, Matt chose "Night in Tunisia" performed by Bud Powell (Gillespie, 1942, Track 4). The song was too cacophonous, although he liked the beat. "Sometimes I don't like jazz at all," he said. This self-observation also reflected his difficulty translating communications that contained dissonance, high volume, or a chaotic context (Knoblauch, 2000). Matt had trouble decoding messages while experiencing stress.

"I have to do things in an orderly manner," he said. "My mind is methodical." He liked robots because they worked and broke in patterned ways.

At the eighth session, Matt wanted to hear classical music. He insisted I choose. We sat quietly, listening to "Glenn Gould and Serenity" (2003). Matt said, "People seem to project things on me. Is that what you call it?" We discussed how he initially assumed everyone perceived him as dark and serious. He said, "Oh that's projection, isn't it? That's how I felt then. Now, no one makes sense." Matt talked about struggling with his parents' divorce when he was 14 years old. It seemed strange they would divorce after so much time together, but he had also anticipated their split due to constant arguing. Matt went to live with his father first. He seldom talked to his mother. "I was more interested in drinking and getting stoned with friends," he said. Marijuana had obstructed his goal, due to a failed drug test at work. He had difficulty seeing the termination of his job as related to his own choice.

In subsequent sessions, Matt selected "Glenn Gould and Serenity" (2003). The music represented an emerging self, a new direction—embracing skilled, technical approaches to emotion. Matt appreciated the music for its technical order, and perhaps unconsciously for the isolation and physical shame it carried as subtext. In a *Psychoanalytic Review* essay, Sperber (1999) delineated the "Cased-In-Man Syndrome" from a constellation of personality traits, typified by Gould. The traits, several of which Matt shared, included: over-controlling and perfectionism, living in a hermit's abode, working with limited human contact, hypersensitivity to ridicule and humiliation, and high sensitivity to constructive criticism due to manipulation by shame in early childhood. Gould biographer, psychiatrist Peter Ostwald (1997), perceived Gould's social withdrawal, isolation, and obsessive attention to ritualized behavior as indicating Asperger's Syndrome.

While listening to Gould, Matt reminisced about his rugby career, as a vehicle for discussing ambivalent feelings about same-gender interpersonal relations. Matt described dislocating a shoulder in a game. He mimicked the "chicken wing pose," an opponent had pulled Matt's arm into during a scrum. Matt had previously dislocated that person's knee. Matt flatly described the mechanical, aggressive interactions involving dominance, defeat, and metaphorical dismemberment. To heal his shoulder, Matt's father taught him to hang from a bar in a doorway until the shoulder popped back. This method symbolized the detachment, lack of nurturing, and inherent humiliation in their relationship. Matt showed how the shoulder still popped out at times. He abruptly ended the session to check on a medication side effect—preferring the quick fix to leaving unsettling memories exposed.

Italian psychiatrists Peccecia and Benedetti (1998) believed schizophrenia was the result of an interaction between neurobiological vulnerabilities, unbearable affect, and a non-cohesive and non-integrated self (Koehler, 2003). They observed a de-integration between the separate and symbiotic selves of the patient resulting in the person moving between pathological symbiosis, or merging with the world, and defensive retreat, in an autistic manner (Koehler, 2003; Peccecia & Benedetti, 1998). This seemed to describe Matt's rough transition into adulthood. He had lost the boundaries between himself and his friends who were exploring their sexuality. Then he retreated until he felt isolated from others.

At the next session, Matt asked for Gluck's (1762, Side 1: Track 4) "Dance of the Blessed Spirits" that he had heard in skills group. After that, he returned to Portishead. The rhythm between merging and isolating that Matt struggled with, and which might challenge ongoing treatment, was sonically captured in Portishead's music. This British soul band that debuted in the

1990s was referred to as trip-hop, because of its intimate, abandoning trance-slow rhythms, and creepy, sorrowful lyrics. The lead singer Beth Gibbons seemed "unhinged" and frightened by her own music (Edna, 2008). The band claimed to be responding musically to an era of stealth politics, deteriorating health care, and wars. In some Portishead songs, sounds battled with other sounds, with no apparent hierarchy, much like schizophrenic patients might experience with numerous competing voices. The band used a soft discord of noises—rotating helicopter blades, computers, and static—to create a foreboding atmosphere (Frere-Jones, 2008).

Given Matt's preference for machines over people, Portishead offered a perfect feast. The song "Mysterons" revolved around, an electronic instrument, a Theremin, that produced spooky wails once popular in old horror films (Ellis, 1995). In Portishead songs, machines and humans ebbed and mixed in stimulating and sedating patterns. Many songs on Portishead's debut album *Dummy* (Gibbons, 1994) focused on guilt and fear. This music aligned with Matt's feelings of paranoia, and ambivalence about the future. Portishead articulated feelings that Matt acted or projected outwards; thus the eerie chorus of voice and machines was likely cathartic.

"I feel like my imagination was better last week," Matt said in a final session. "Today I see things clearly but with less color. The world's duller." He feared returning to a dissociative place, the stone precipice of his own serious face. Within the space an iPod and music allowed, Matt had discussed homoerotic urges, aggression and feelings of revenge toward his own masochism. Intimacy, for Matt, was in things and gestures, and more gradually, in people.

It is not surprising that Matt's psychosis accompanied a persistent use of cannabis and alcohol. The disinhibition he experienced when using substances made him more vulnerable to psychosis (Arendt, Rosenberg, Foldager, Perto, & Munk-Jørgensen, 2005). Once Matt's emotions awoke, he became steadily overwhelmed, until destroying the machine of himself seemed less painful than the prospect of being illogical (Charles, 2002). Matt described the cuts on his arms as attention seeking. He intellectualized to keep his suicide attempt out of awareness.

Matt seemed to develop an ability to better tolerate silence. He gradually allowed music, rather than monologue or dialogue, to fill the void. Matt and I developed a rapport, despite, and because of ruptures and repairs. He employed me as a messy-haired mirror with whom he practiced interpersonal responses. He felt safe while listening to music together. He did not want disorganized input and murky mirroring from other patients. At the final session, Matt asked that I keep his Portishead music in mind—thus to stay in attunement with him.

Elliot, first introduced in chapter 3, was more difficult to establish rapport with than Matt. Elliot was suspicious of medications, and adamant that an emotionally numb life was intolerable—a conviction that Theuma, Read, Moscowitz, and Stewart (2007) say is common to young adults. Elliot was a highly sensitive young man whose older siblings were high achievers. Accepting and complying with medications was akin to living in dispassionate exile, which his parents (and I, at the time) hoped he would choose. An embattled pattern of individuation and dependency, and of trust and mistrust, echoed throughout his hospital stay.

Like Matt, Elliot linked emotional expressions to music. After hearing a Bach cello piece (1717–1723) performed by Yo-Yo Ma Elliot said, "I hate the lethargic, bored way medicine makes me feel. My mind is usually sharp. It bothers me everyone wants me on medication." I ruptured our link as noted previously by intellectualizing his feelings. En route back to his room, I fumbled at a locked door. I had disorganized feelings when passing with Elliot through real and metaphorical transitions. Our connection never found a steady rhythm again.

Elliot allowed there to be a brief link between us while we listened to Radiohead's "Nude" (Yorke & Greenwood, 2007, Track 3). He talked about a Radiohead concert he had attended on a rainy August eve. He said, "I remember the day of the concert and how complete I felt. I wish you had been there. The rain was falling with the music."

Radiohead was named the ideal voice for a generation of young nihilists like Elliot, obsessed with zombies and the apocalypse (Binelli, 2008; Bronfman, 2008). Radiohead's music was full of false starts and dissonances reflecting the chaos of modern life (Binelli, 2008). The band focused on love, death, despair, rage, and dread that life and illness would wear us down (Pareles, 2007, Gordon, 2003). Radiohead's lead singer, Tom Yorke, was an avatar for Elliot. Yorke's voice brandished hot and cold intimacy, a yearning that seduced listeners along with a detachment that shunned them (Pareles, 2007). In working with Elliot's ambivalence about intimacy, a clinician would benefit from learning Elliot's opening and closing rhythms. With Elliot, I experienced self-doubt when subjected to the cold eye Elliot turned on himself.

At a later session, Elliot turned to Tool's songs to accompany explanations of how he felt altered by mania or depression. "It does scare me that I get too manic and I want something—a pill—to take," he said. I mentioned lifestyle changes and how hard it must be to face decisions about medications at Elliot's young age. He agreed. Together, we devised an analogy of how being drafted into military service would equally, drastically change a person's life. There seemed to be tentative repair, but I missed the delicate rhythm of attunement a second time by mentioning how Elliot could negotiate medications with a physician. Elliot looked up suddenly as if someone were standing behind me: "I thought I heard my mother's voice," he said.

Elliot had heard in my voice the critical tone his parents used; his sensitive ear caught all levels of communication (Knoblauch, 2000), even the ones I had not owned then.

At the next session, Elliot was dismissive which stimulated countertransference feelings of failing him (Searles, 1979). "What did you download?" he asked. He wanted to listen to music without talking. He was polite, but his body language (i.e., crossed arms, lack of eye contact) was defensive. He was tired of talking about and studying emotions. He selected Rolling Stones' (Jagger & Richards, 1973, Track 5) "Angie." "I have impressions of a lost love. I want to keep those to myself," he said. Elliot described "closed and cynical," feelings in response to Jagger that he linked to his love of Conrad's (1902) novella "Heart of Darkness." Conrad's description of Kurtz's unraveling mind paralleled for Elliot his retreat into the urban forests of Stanley Park.

Elliot had a fantasy that Jagger wrote Angie when he was Elliot's age; this fantasy heightened Elliot's feelings of twinship with Jagger (Spotnitz, 2004). Jagger cherished an identity that rebelled against the status quo, while also conforming to its pragmatism and hierarchies. Jagger was a walking human conflict, but unlike Elliot, he had the capacity to contain and exploit these contradictions. He was patriarchal and feminine, energetic and passive, cruel and tender (Cox, 1990). Elliot was caught in the gap between becoming a surgeon or a sound engineer and between grieving a female lover and trying to kiss a male friend.

Jagger created personas that fit the lyrics of each song he sang (Palmer, 1987). Elliot's efforts to create identity were undermined by strong need states and hypersensitivity. Elliot found refuge for vulnerable feelings in Jagger's aloofness. Even when Jagger was tender, such as in a rare ballad like "Angie" (Jagger & Richards, 1973, Track 5), the singer walked away unscathed. Jagger was the choreographer, not the victim, of break-ups. Elliot wanted to be Jagger-like, focusing on technical aspects of music and love. He made more sense of himself within the context of a Rolling Stones, Radiohead, or Tool song rather than being reduced to an illness identity. Music was the one territory wherein Elliot could preserve a sense of agency.

Elliot's and other participants' observations about music seemed to align at times with the survey results from researchers who gathered data on patients survey to gather data from patients with psychosis about music and music therapy in their treatment. Participants reported that music offered freedom in taking their minds off illness; freedom from stigma through sharing their tastes, interests, and musical abilites; freedom from "illness centered" treatment, contact with one's self and inner core; contact with aliveness and bodily awareness; and contact with emotions through paying attention, expression, and creativity (Solli & Rolvsjord, 2015).

Seneca was the third young adult whose psychosis seemed born, even more than Elliot's, out of the rave scene. Seneca struggled with illicit drugs and early schizophrenia. Seneca was compact and graceful like a gymnast, with a Mohawk strip of purple hair. From the first day Seneca arrived at the psychiatric hospital—singing a love ballad—until the day he left for the state hospital, his illness worsened. In addition to being literally locked up on a psychiatric unit, Seneca was locked up metaphorically inside an extended dissociative state. The strongest cocktail of antipsychotics could not penetrate his psychotic shell. The one thing that reached through to Seneca—and what he reached back through—was music. Some of Seneca's music selections seemed enfolded and encoded in his substance use history and fragmentation. This leads to the question of whether music may sometimes trigger rumination in patients with psychosis, and how a clinician could help bring that into a patient's awareness.

Seneca initially listened at the door while I worked with other patients. Sometimes he would brush past me in the hall, his arm grazing mine, or he would stand in close proximity until I turned. He would quickly retreat when discovered. In some ways, Seneca seemed like a vigilant and stealth feral cat: drawing close, then pulling away. There was an ebb and flow to the angles of Seneca's intimacy (Ready, 2013).

San Francisco, the mecca of the West Coast rave scene, was the center of Seneca's world. His social identity and his fantasy of an idealized family were forged in rave culture. That's also where Seneca began using salvia divinorum, an unrestricted herb grown in the Oaxaca region of Mexico (Giroud, Felber, Augsburger, Horisberger, Rivier & Mangin, 2000). An article in *The American Journal of Psychiatry* (Prezekop & Lee, 2009) presented the case of a twenty-one-year-old man with no psychiatric history who came to a hospital with symptoms of acute psychosis; he was highly agitated and paranoid. Prezekop and Lee (2009) concluded that the young man was predisposed to schizophrenia, but that salvia divinorum—which influences brain dopamine levels and potentiates plastic changes in frontal lobe networks—precipitated the young man's psychotic break. He was unresponsive to strong doses of antipsychotic medications.

Cannabis, which Seneca started using in early adolescence, has been considered another instigator of schizophrenia (Hall, 1998). A study in Denmark indicated that approximately half the people hospitalized for cannabis-induced psychosis would be diagnosed subsequently with schizophrenia spectrum disorders (Arendt et al., 2005). There seems to be a higher risk of developing schizophrenia for someone genetically vulnerable to that illness if cannabis is used at an earlier age (Cohen, Solowiji, & Carr, 2008). Researchers have speculated that 14 percent of psychotic outcomes in young people would not have occurred if cannabis had not been consumed (Henquet et. al., 2005; Moore, Zammit, Lignford-Hughes, et al., 2007).

From the first session, Seneca did not ask for special downloaded music. He was focused on attuning to my music, just as I was focused on attuning to his. Searles (1979) observed that "the more ill a patient is, the more deeply indispensable does he need to become, at a pre-individuation level of ego functioning to his transference-mother." Seneca, like Elliot, shifted between linking through musical selections and attacking links in a manner described by Bion (1959/1984a). Seneca would abruptly leave the room, or choose misogynistic songs.

One particularly poignant moment of connection with Seneca occurred while we listened together to Tool. I arrived at that session tired and irritable, which seemed to allow me to align with the music's primal anger. I was surprised to find the music soothing. I sensed a silent attunement with Seneca, which arrived with a sense of dread. I stared intently at the iPod and speaker as if those objects might—or as if they did—slide across the table. I wondered about Seneca's unsettling psychic processes. During that session, Seneca seemed to be navigating between joining with me in symbiosis and being stuck in autistic isolation (Pececcia & Benedetti, 2005; Koehler, 2003). Seneca remained resident in my psyche long after that music listening session ended. Working with him required revisiting personal memories of childhood fragmentation and psychological precipices. When Seneca was abruptly discharged to the state hospital, I felt a sense of urgency about sending him a music CD. It is still unclear to me whether I was trying to save Seneca or myself from hopelessness about cracks and holes in the mental health system.

Young adults like Seneca, Matt, and Elliot live in a modern world that does not match nature's rhythms in them. To survive a highly anxious age, a person must tune himself to various distortions of sound. Those who are more sensitive and responsive to new sound technologies may need more guidance, to hold their own rhythm in a dissonant world. Containment and expression through music for a person with psychosis may be a process of gradual attunement and mutual awareness in the company of an also listening clinician.

It is important to note here that music has its dark side. As we have witnessed in this chapter, music can become intimately entwined with, and even incite urges for, substance use. Music—combined with cannabis, alcohol, or with emerging designer drugs—can help stimulate early psychosis and fragmentation. We have intimated in earlier chapters, that music is addictive, and may suspend a person within a complex of linked addictions. Some patients have negative associations with music, or find it overstimulating (as we will discuss in chapter 8) so that it is impossible to use in conjunction with clinical work. For other patients, drug memories and addictive cravings are activated by certain pieces of music, which tap into the brain reward system (Fachner, 2010). Listening to music with a clinician may help the patient learn how to be in the here and now, and experience the music in an unaltered self-state, thus creating a new explicit way to approach a song.

I'm aware that music can also be a soundtrack, and motivating force for horrific acts. The same Wagnerian music that saved my uncle's life is a source of despair for individuals and families impacted by the Holocaust who associate that composer's music with anti-Semitism and Hitler. As Plato (1970) warned, music can serve as a force for destructive social interactions such as riots or violent acts against women. Working with music in one's self and with others, and thus working in the realm of memory, metaphor, and emotion, is complex.

Chapter 7

Wrote on Your Wall Before Leaving

I never listened to music with Alyssa; I never met her. She rented a studio a few doors down from a journalist friend. Before the night Alyssa fell from her window ledge, she had posted several entries on Facebook about childhood sexual abuse. She wrote, "Thanks everyone for your concern. I had a rather emotional breakthrough regarding molesting that happened in my past. I've dealt with it and you should hope to see really great things from me" (Frizzelle, 2012). A few days later, she posted: "I'm dealing with things. Maybe we could start a chat group for people who have been through this experience." This was followed by an entry in which she offered to give coping tools to other molestation survivors. She suggested people message her privately or post on the comment section of her page (Frizzelle, 2012).

This chapter is a fantasy and a case study about potential uses of music to build rapport and establish human connection—with people on the brink of suicide. It is possible that music as gesture and tool could help a person in crisis contain overwhelming feelings and metabolize trauma. Music, beginning with an authentic, empathic voice might help a person tolerate intense affective states, including emptiness, until the threat of self-harm has passed. I am also asking us to ponder the importance of making a cultural shift toward mental health recovery—wherein we consider the perspective of a person experiencing psychosis (which may have been born out of trauma) and how we could engage, include, and listen to her within our communities (Davidson, Tondora, Lawless, O'Connell, & Rowe, 2009).

Emergency rooms and psychiatric hospitals have become central portals where re-enacted traumas are received (Owens et al., 2010; Szegedy-Maszak, 2004). As this trend increases, we will need to discover what hospital best practices might calm rather than re-stimulate trauma for vulnerable patients. At the same time, we could bolster health professionals who may become vicariously traumatized while providing triage treatments for patients in disorganized states. In the midst of layers of chaos, how do professionals hold steady in transitional spaces? In high-stress environments like acute psychiatric hospitals, safe rapport may need to be built within the brief span of one song, or in the gesture of one pink geranium or one calming voice. We clinicians sometimes bear witness to a terrible internal dissonance of abandonment.

We uncover Seneca's clues left where language has been undone, or decode Anna's gestural narratives of abuse. Alyssa, who inspired this chapter, re-enacted an earlier traumatic scene through a suicidal gesture—what Ferenczi (1929) called "an aversion to life acquired at a young age," or "the confusion of being a sexual being before a sexual age" (p. 127).

Alyssa had recently relocated from Alaska. The journalist who lived a few doors down encountered her for the first time when he heard screams coming from her apartment late one night. He found other neighbors gathered in the hallway outside Alyssa's door. Earlier, when two neighbors had knocked, Alyssa, wearing only underwear, opened the door wide enough for them to see her face and body caked in white powder. Powder also covered her floors. Ghostly footsteps on the hallway carpet were later discovered to be traces of flour (Frizzelle, 2012).

The two neighbors compared glimpses of information. Alyssa had apparently been carrying a white bag. Inside the bag was a white cat, which she had stabbed with a kitchen knife. "The cat is out of the bag," she told the young neighbors. "I have killed it." When they asked what, she replied "Me." She explained that she was from the future and had returned to fetch something. She asked them to call her boyfriend, then slammed the door (Frizzelle, 2012).

Alyssa seemed to be re-enacting the agony of a traumatic experience as Winnicott (1974) described in his concept of the fear of a breakdown that has already happened. Alyssa looked to the future for details from the past that would emerge to clarify the shadowy story of her molestation. She may not have actually experienced her original abuse due to dissociation or to lack of sufficient ego structure to process the devastating event (Winnicott, 1974, pp. 103–107).

Alyssa's psychotic episode pushed the re-enactment of a brutal scene out into the environment. She performed the already-experienced death of her innocence and the destruction of her child psyche through her ghostly appearance and the symbol of her bleeding white cat. Alyssa's neighbors were thrown into chaos by the bizarre, violent scene. The neighbor who dialed 911 paused when asked, "Is this an emergency?" (Frizzelle, 2012). Was it? What words could she have used then to convey the delicate, tenuous nature of the primitive scene she had witnessed? The police arrived with sirens blaring.

They broke Alyssa's door down after knocking with no response. Alyssa greeted them sitting on her windowsill. Then folded forward from her sixth-floor window.

Later, we learned that Alyssa had been fired from a sex supply emporium and a pizza restaurant. She volunteered at a medical marijuana dispensary. Her behaviors leading up to the suicide had been increasingly manic and erratic, alienating her boyfriend and friends.

Even these brief snapshots reveal Alyssa's struggles with feeling unwanted—by employers and her romantic partner—which reignited feelings of hopelessness. Asking for help at a time of crisis can be complicated. How would Alyssa describe, so that a listener could apprehend, the feeling of what Bion (1984) called being physically assaulted, or murdered by one's own dangerous emotions? Moreover, how could she express such a complex feeling when she herself had not yet grasped the feeling? How does a young, fragile person both hide and reveal a dark secret, with its inherent accompanying wish to be saved, without destroying herself? Alyssa first tried to appeal to other molestation survivors on Facebook by offering to display other people's painful stories, while desperately needing safe containment for her own.

Kierkegaard (1954) noted that the self is a synthesis in which the finite is the limiting factor and the infinite is the expanding factor; the despair inherent in infinitude was "the fantastical, the limitless" (p. 181). A suicide's communication of despair may include the terror of being trapped inside an unbounded implicit moment, which expands into an unending future. At the same time, the person feels locked up within a self without boundaries. That undefined self can enter other forms, or be entered from anywhere.

It's unclear what nexus of events incited Alyssa's traumatic memory of abuse to emerge . . . the break-up, the lost job, or isolation in a new city? What is also unclear is the role dis-inhibiting substances played in her management of unsettling memories? Alyssa could not bear the weight of emerging feelings. She pushed her sense impressions back out into the environment through what Bion (1984) has described as symbolic, ritual behaviors that for Alyssa involved cleansing, sacrificing, masking, and transforming. It is not clear that Alyssa wanted to die. What is certain is her need, even unconsciously, to communicate.

Michael Eigen (1993) in "The Psychotic Core" noted that unintegration—which Winnicott (1953) viewed as leading to fragmentation and Bion saw as a deformed and deforming container, can be both disturbing and renewing. The story of Alyssa seems to move in what Eigen saw as a human pattern, between the more manic state of believing all things are possible (Facebook support) to the depressive state of seeing nothing as possible (on the ledge). Eigen also underscores the importance of the clinician holding out hope for the transformative potential of what has fallen apart coming back together. He notes the terror one experiences in psychosis as a fluid impending sense of annihilation and rigidity like a "suffocating trap" (p. 348).

I wonder how a clinically minded person could have engaged sufficiently with Alyssa to gain brief trust, and lightly emotionally scaffold her with enough ventilation not to frighten her. Could an emergency responder have approached in a less aggressive manner—by entering through her window, or talking to her through her door? Would it have helped if a first responder had foreknowledge of Alyssa's struggles with the ghostly intrusion of unsettling memories? I suspect that the use of music, prior to that moment and in that moment might have provided an immediate, non-verbal, affective connection. Such speculation is useless, except to consider in a moment, the importance of an abiding humane urge to connect. Writer Andy Bodle (2014) printed an essay in "The Guardian" about being saved from suicide by hearing a random Phil Collins song he later came to dislike.

A musically attuned therapist might have detected Alyssa's ambivalence toward life before she ever began her ritual re-enactment. Researchers (Ozdas, Shiavi, Wilkes, Silverman, & Silverman, 2004) have identified common vocal features somewhat similar to those noted in depression for people who were pre-suicidal, including loss of energy, and power, and monotonous repetitious, and uninflected speech. Voices were hollow and toneless as though the person were lacking a center. The researchers also noticed a decrease in harmonic overtones and resonance (a lack of anxious patterns) in people at risk for suicide and concurred that a pre-suicidal voice patterning was a unique pathological configuration.

Insight into the musical qualities of the human voice under various states of distress could be useful in establishing urgent connections with patients experiencing psychosis, or caught in delusional re-enactments. Equally useful for clinicians and mental health professionals would be an ability to attune to the rhythms of their own "embodied countertransferences" to help detect when patients were in danger and help regulate patients when possible. McDougall (1986) described attending in therapy to the patient's body which does not speak a language but which frames the psychic scenes of the patient's internal world, including preverbal trauma.

In Andrew Solomon's *The Noonday Demon* (2001), the author cited three groups of people who attempt suicide. The first group he described—driven to desperation by pain fatigue—attempt suicide as an act of exorcism (Alvarez, 1971). This would seem to describe Alyssa's attempt to sacrifice the damaged part of herself that had been previously sacrificed through sexual abuse. Fairbairn (1952) believed that psychotherapists were the "true successors to the exorcist" focused on "forgiveness of sins and the casting out of devils" (p. 70) and thus were the ideal people to interpret suicidal gestures.

I would add that in order to aid an expedient attunement where trust is tenuous or has been subsumed by trauma, the most effective human connection might be indirect—such as one facilitated by a simple melody.

Among Solomon's (2001) the second group are people driven toward suicide as if it were an ambition without the constraints of ambition. Inherent in this group would be someone who attempts suicide as an act of anger. A well-timed intervention, such as through music or some other connecting mechanism, might divert or help sublimate lethal urges. Musical works by Lil Wayne, Beethoven, or Metallica might help structure the expression of rage or help to release the pressure and heat of anger. One young woman who came to the hospital had carefully burned a series of CDs for her friends and family filled with music that conveyed her pain and frustration. None of her closest friends, nor her therapist, decoded her clues. Her next attempt to communicate involved a handful of pills and driving her car into a wall.

Pragmatists were Solomon's (2001) third group: they followed a line of faulty logic to conclude that death would provide escape from intolerable problems. Solomon noticed a common denominator with this group of a history of trauma, suicide, and childhood loss mixed with a chronic inability to process that loss or any other grief. In such cases might listening together to a gospel song by Betty Levette, a Chet Baker solo, or a Chopin piano prelude facilitate the containment of overwhelming emotions in both patient and clinician. One suicidal patient processed his grief about the loss of his family and identity by talking about and tuning in to Delilah's radio broadcasts. The nationally syndicated radio host focuses on creating community around sharing and soothing listeners' emotional pain (Ready, 2014). Music has such vast capacity to hold, digest, and transport emotions. Bion (1984) noted the importance of a clinician framing her own affect to be better posed to help a patient metabolize pain. Music is a potentially strong cornerstone of a therapeutic frame as well as a mediator of affect in a crisis.

Numerous writers, including Solomon (2012), have described a sense of meaningless in the modern world wherein psychic victims embody existing gaps in social fabric. What drives suicidal people toward desperate ledges may also involve oppressive or restrictive aspects of a society (Durkheim, 2006). Unspoken traumas could cause a person to experience an inner world invaded by annihilation anxiety and terror. The person could feel abandoned as an isolated other, a rejected object, and without community or cultural connections, which could describe the cases of Alyssa, Anna, or Seneca, among others. Contemporary American society has few built-in mechanisms to help reintegrate people who experience trauma or psychosis. We meet ritual re-enactments like Alyssa's with a show of force, or a defensive urgency.

In hindsight, it seems possible that a number of linked approaches might help clinicians engage with a person, like Alyssa, experiencing strong urges toward suicide. Approaching with a consistent tone of voice attuned to matching, and even providing counterpoint is useful, or approaching with soothing or cathartic music, or even exploring the metaphoric aspects of meaningful music with patients. In times of crisis, or in working with acutely disturbed patients, it is often hard for clinicians and other mental health professionals to hold our minds steady. Music may be the clinical tool whose metaphoric qualities slowly help metabolize a patient's intense projections of terror and dread? My fantasy regarding Alyssa is that she wanted a witness: she wanted to be embraced in her performance of suffering, rather than being marginalized or missed again. Jung (1969/1928) observed that the abreaction of trauma was less healing for patients than the rehearsal of a negative experience in the presence of a clinician. A clinically minded witness could help observe and validate the otherness, as a gesture toward inviting reintegration (Kalshed, 1996, p. 67). What might have unfolded differently if a clinically minded person had ritually received the wounded cat, or become the compassionate witness Alyssa searched for on Facebook?

This brings us back to observing social portals and contexts, within which we receive suicidal gestures and re-enactments. The Facebook promise of connection might result in a disappointing illusion. Unless a person has established a Facebook persona close to an authentic self, or has already solidified relationships of sufficient depth with online friends, then desperate cries for help, cached inside positive aphorisms, will likely not be decoded. Alyssa's proximal neighbors several doors down had no idea she was so desperate.

If Alyssa had been coaxed away from the ledge during her psychotic episode, she would have been transported to an acute psychiatric hospital, on a seventy-two-hour involuntarily hold. There, Alyssa would have been provided with a bed, a diagnosis, and a variety of medications to address symptoms. She would be safely contained without knives, paper clips, or strings on her sweatshirts. Her suicidal gesture would remain unexamined. Psychiatric hospitals are more akin to quarantine camps, where people decompress after isolation in states of extreme anguish or anhedonia. The details of Alyssa's crisis (the white powder and the sacrificed cat) would be precisely noted on hospital forms and court documents. Given Alyssa's fragile psychological state, she would likely have experienced hospitalization as re-traumatizing, with locked doors, unfamiliar protocols, forced medications, and the collective disorganization of other patients.

Freud and Jung (in Kalshed, 1996) agreed that the memory of a traumatic event was often confabulated with unconscious fantasies—making it hard to distinguish fact from fiction, and thus worsening trauma. What if psychiatric hospitals employed aesthetic means to address trauma, through helping patients to transform or transcend the experience, and through helping patients and staff reintegrate traumatic experience through performance or production. The desire to act out a ritual, distinct from an everyday routine, may be a key aspect of a suicide attempt.

I am advocating here the importance of music as one of several possible aesthetic, symbolic rituals in the process of healing trauma, both for those who have experienced trauma, and for the professionals who care for them. Santayana (1955) noted that art does not seek out the pathetic, the tragic, and the absurd; life imposes them on our attention and enlists art in their service (p. 136). He believed art made the contemplation of inevitable tragedy tolerable. Our need to translate trauma into a ritual may be as innate in us as the urge to sing, or the depiction of a hunt on the wall of a Pleistocene cave. We may be wired to practice healing trauma together, just as in lower Manhattan we have the opportunity to practice grief at the site of two solemn black fountains.

Thus far, we have noted how attuned connection, containment, and shared expression of emotion between a clinician and patient can help foster the healing process. A beloved song or a ritualized dance performance can be witnessed and shared in a transitional space that allows interplay between environment, emotions, and senses. We will return to the story of Alyssa after we consider the case of Manu, for whom music was a useful tool in helping to process inner conflicts that led to his suicide attempt. Manu was a willowy young Pacific Islander staying in the US on a work visa. He took an overdose of pills soon after his first consensual homosexual encounter. Suicide was an attempt to split off and exorcise the offensive, gay part of himself, which he could not easily integrate into his strict Catholic childhood and culture.

Manu had immediately confessed his homosexual liaison to his female manager, Carmen, at the fast-food restaurant where he worked. Besides being his boss, Carmen was Manu's landlord, and a surrogate mother figure. She was also his lover. Carmen fired Manu and threw him out of her apartment. Her anger and incredulity at Manu's sexual "transgression" paralleled Manu's anticipated rejection by his Catholic mother. The dreaded loss of his mother, who was adamantly anti-gay, and the actual loss of his benefactor-mother, Carmen, overwhelmed Manu. At the same time, Manu struggled with the emergence of distressing childhood memories of ritual sexual exploitation by an uncle. Manu had kept the molestation a secret since the 4th grade, when the illicit events began occurring. He had also avoided addressing sexual identity issues, likely hoping to escape internal conflict by moving to a new country.

Manu did not have enough psychological structure, or sufficient resources, to accommodate the unbearable stress of "socialization ambiguity" (McDade & Worthman, 2004). He was caught between conflicting expectations crashing into desires, a pattern identified by Mageo (2008). He lived in a shifting crevasse between polar opposites. His mood swung from anxious/manic to depressed/defeated while he was in the hospital. He moved equally rapidly between straight and queer orientations. He longed to be the obedient son, and he wanted to reinvent himself as an independent urban gangster. Manu also had a strong urge to dance, although he was exceedingly shy.

One challenge of working with Manu was to manage countertransference urges to save him. Manu would seem to disappear or get lost. He asked others to make decisions for him—even to guide his sexual orientation. Language was also a barrier. Manu had trouble with language translation when delusional or confused. When we communicated through music, particularly when working with the voices of his three favorite musicians—Jason Derulo, Lil Wayne, and Michael Jackson—Manu was better able to organize himself. The music and musicians embodied a transitional space within which Manu could explore various aspects of his fragmented identity. His lost and lonely feelings had begun long before he came to the US.

When Manu arrived at the hospital, he was caught in a process of "splitting" (Freud, 1933/1964; Klein, 1948; Grotstein, 1981), and at the conjunction of a number of intra-psychic and interpersonal conflicts. He had moved to America, like many young Pacific Islanders, to earn money to send home to his family (MacPherson, 1994; O'Meara, 1990). Manu encountered instead a failing US economy that offered minimal opportunities. In recent years, European and North American researchers have studied the impact of migration, social adversity, urbanicity, and globalization on psychosis. Several studies of immigrants and ethnic groups in multicultural societies have linked aspects of the acculturation experience to negative behavioral, psychological, and somatic symptoms (Berry, Kim, Minde, & Mok, 1987; Hovey & King, 1996; Krishnan & Berry, 1992; Liebkind, 1996; Montgomery, 1992; Sam & Berry, 1995).

Manu, Alyssa, and Harika all experienced displacement and social defeat—a concept from animal studies. Social defeat refers to the effects of an animal (or a person) being dominated in a contest or interaction (Cantor-Graae, 2007; Luhrmann, 2007). Sustained stress from social defeat may lead to alterations in the central nervous system in terms of dopamine sensitivity and regulating the dopaminergic system, thus causing vulnerability to psychosis (Cantor-Graae 2007; Selten & Cantor-Graae, 2004).

Manu was so hypersensitive to sensory and interpersonal stimulation that I wondered whether he had experienced a reactive psychotic episode due to lack of social support, and no coping resources. We are still coming to terms with how globalization, the high-tech revolution, and social change are impacting the mental health of young people throughout the world (Schoeffel, 2000; Thornton, Kerslake, Binns, 2010). Young men who move away from small villages to urban areas seeking work often indulge in new, non-traditional freedoms, without having the internal ego structure to handle the consequences of rapid changes (Holmes, 1983).

Manu was a young man standing on a metaphoric ledge who seemed, as had Elliot, to benefit from musical role models and beloved music as launching platforms for psychological exploration. One of Manu's favorite musicians, Jason Derulo, was a Haitian-American pop singer, born in Florida, who debuted on *American Idol* after having studied music, dance, and acting (Brown, 2009; 2010). Derulo served as a mirror for the ego image Manu wanted to embody (Spotnitz, 2004): the "good" immigrant embraced by postcolonial culture. In addition, the idealized Derulo-self was the hopeful image Manu wanted to portray to his family. In attempting to exorcise the traumatized object—the abused self–Manu opened the door to embody a different aspect of the immigrant role. With Derulo as our soundtrack, we began our music listening sessions, talking about the challenges of offering his mother financial support and his fantasies about a successful life in the US. Manu spoke about his abuse, and confused emotions of anger and love for his uncle and for the difficulties of daily US life.

Lil Wayne better symbolized another side of Manu's split: the angry other's voice. Like Derulo, Lil Wayne followed a modified golden road through the music industry starting as a teen. His trajectory trailed through darker skies. At the time that Manu was in the hospital, Lil Wayne was serving an eight-month sentence for illegal gun possession at Rikers Island (Eligon, 2010). In Manu's preferred song, "Drop The World" (Carter, 2009, Track 8), Lil Wayne expressed rebellion against oppression and frustrated anger about the elusiveness of success in a beleaguered environment. Wayne gave voice to the rage and disillusionment of young people struggling with social defeat. When Manu listened to Lil Wayne, his demeanor shifted from submissive politeness to anger; he was able to think more clearly about a future.

Manu's other frequent musical choice was Michael Jackson, who embodied various psychological splits (Baldwin, 1998). Unlike Derulo, Jackson embodied the reviled as well as the cherished "other" of American culture. Jackson expressed and embodied Manu's ambivalence about committing to a culture, a sexual orientation, a persona, or even to life itself. Listening to Jackson with Manu allowed us to abide in and tolerate together the metaphorical cultural spaces that Manu was trying to grasp. Jackson described the unconscious gap within which we could locate such dialectics as sane and mad, dark-skinned and white, fantasy and reality, male and female, and gay and straight. Jackson accomplished this delicate balancing feat in the context of melodic, accessible music. He concretized and memorialized ambivalence in a manner that allowed listeners to embrace ambivalence and dance toward momentary transcendence of the pain of embodiment with its suffering.

While listening to Manu's favorite music, we talked about events influencing Manu's overdose. He was more present in the company of music, allowing anger to surface when an artist invited anger into the room. I wondered, reflecting on Manu's progress, how Alyssa might have benefited from a witness and a vicarious voice. Narrative and artistic exploration are pivotal tools in the metabolization and reintegration of traumatic experience. Davoine and Gaudillière (2004) described "societies in which art is medicine" wherein multiple traditions, ceremonial and artistic, bring onstage what cannot be uttered. Health is performed. Music is a useful form of aesthetic experience when working with individuals who have experienced, and who may be re-enacting, trauma. Discerning truth can also be performed; in the reconciliation of internal and external realities, performance brings new meanings into awareness (Aldridge & Fachner, 2006).

If we learn to embrace traumatic communications through the help of aesthetic vehicles, perhaps we can learn to welcome, rather than avoid, the trauma that dwells next door to us. After Alyssa's death, Internet comments focused on her cat, which survived. The cat, as wounded embodiment of Alyssa, transcends this story, just as the anticipating future embracing a dread of the past (Winnicott, 1974) returns to speak to us, traumatized, white as a ghost, asking for a safe place to rest.

Chapter 8

Play Marshall Mathers, Please

Ted, a forty-nine-year-old gay man, had struggled with mental health issues prior to receiving an HIV/AIDS diagnosis. He was gravely disabled, had lost vision in both eyes, and suffered from dementia. Ted usually remained withdrawn from other patients; he seldom spoke more than a few words. His paranoid notions that people wanted to destroy him led to striking out at apparitions, and at hospital staff.

When Ted started attending process groups, he interacted with peers while dancing to 70s and 80s pop music. His movements were precarious and ambling. As he continued to dance, it was possible to catch glimpses of a younger, vibrant Ted socializing in gay bars in an era when his beloved songs, and Ted, were in their prime. Ted rarely expressed anger at having been betrayed and abandoned by friends and family after his AIDS diagnosis. If directly asked about grief, or regret, Ted would say "Oh no, my friends were lovely. My mother cared for me." According to his chart, these statements reflected an idealized fantasy rather than the solitary reality he had faced.

During one music group, Ted became tearful when the jazz standard "Someone to Watch Over Me" (Gershwin & Gershwin, 1926, Track 2) played. He left mid-song to meet with his physician. I offered to play the whole song for Ted once the group had finished. He was uncomfortable sitting with me in a small room. Once the last bars of the song resolved, Ted bolted from the room. He reacted in a similar way when Scott Joplin's "The Entertainer" (1902/2003, Track 4), which he had requested, played. His grandparents, he said, had old ragtime records he had cherished and lost.

Ted did not like to remain among others after demonstrations of emotional vulnerability. He would talk candidly during process group, and then abruptly deny what he had just said. Listeners were left confused, as if holding on to pieces of a torn letter. Ted did not want to be seen or found and yet, without warning, in the middle of a beloved song, when the focus was not directly on him, he would suddenly softly speak about the song's meaning for him.

In this chapter, I will further explore the dynamics of using music as an adjunct therapeutic tool. I will explore how clinicians might employ music in private practice or in group or community settings. In addition, I will explore using music with patients who are experiencing various mental health conditions such as PTSD, major depressive disorder, and personality disorders. For people experiencing serious mental health issues, listening to music with a caring professional (rather than in isolation) can renew social connections, as well as help reconstruct narratives to include more restorative associations. The beauty of shared listening experiences involves an indirect focus on interpersonal interactions. A more direct approach might feel too exposing, thus prohibitive, for the patient.

Without music, it is hard to imagine that Harika or Anna would have continued meeting for any sustained amount of time with a clinician. The dynamics of why this musical mode of connectivity is effective is well supported by neurological research and early infancy research where preverbal communications between mother and infant are described in musical terms (Trevarthen, 1999; Trevarthen & Malloch, 2000).

Listening to music with patients inside the stark environment of an acute psychiatric hospital differs from listening to music in a private practice setting designed to encourage calm and containment. In a psychiatric hospital, Lil Wayne's "Drop The World" (Carter, 2009, Track 8) or Johnny Cash's "Folsom Prison Blues" can provide empathic witness to confirm a wordless rage. Such songs effectively metabolize anger for patients frustrated by involuntary detainment, or abandoned by family. Kohut (1957) noted the potency of the music's cathartic potential: "Musical experience (especially by 'oral' listening) may . . . relieve a person's deepest tension anxieties (and thus secondarily, diminish his frustrated raging) by permitting the regressive experience of a primitive narcissistic equilibrium" (p. 8). Listening to music with lyrics allows for additional benefits, such as the introduction of metaphors, upon which a patient can elaborate, but which he is not pressured to invent. Harika focused on angels, Matt's music and conversation emphasized machines as a metaphor. One patient, Betty, whose terminal cancer led to increased psychotic episodes, exchanged cereal boxes for song selections that pleased her; she stacked single serving boxes of Corn Flakes and Fruit Loops next to the iPod, saying, "Eat, you are thin," thus reversing the metabolization process, providing nourishment, whenever a song touched her.

Patients who have easy access to smart phones, MP3 players, and music streaming applications like Pandora have an ongoing, dynamic relationship with music. They use music, albeit not always with conscious intent, for relaxation, for expression, for distraction, or even for changing or affirming a mood. If we introduce a music listening device into the therapeutic dyad or a group setting, the music device becomes an intrinsic part of creating and maintaining the potential space (Hug & Lohne, 2009). We have already discussed how patients like Ted may prefer to give and receive information without intense, direct therapeutic focus on them. A device playing music can embody a third-person perspective in therapy; music also activates areas of the brain that help integrate narrative and sensory emotional information processing, and thus could be supportive of talk therapy (Decety & Chaminade, 2005; Ruby & Decety, 2001).

The iPod as a tangible object containing familiar music can be an accessible co-facilitator assisting in something akin to the alpha function (Bion, 1967/1984) when working with hard-to-reach patients. Perhaps, more precisely, it is the composer or artist who performs their process of metabolizing raw beta elements of emotions into structured alpha material for the patient that we can witness.

James, a young African-American man, would stop me each day in the hallway to ask if I would please play Eminem, though he always used the musician's birth name—Marshall Mathers. James had been diagnosed with psychosis, NOS; he suffered from command hallucinations that urged him toward suicide. I wondered if his voices, which seemed to him to rap in strident anger, were unified under the voice of Eminem. The singer was known for organizing random scribblings on small pieces of paper, scraps of rhyming couplets that turned a chaos of thoughts into an ordered and replicable form. Eminem's manager compared his client to John Nash, the Nobel Prize–winning economist who struggled with schizophrenia (Caramanica, 2008). Eminem was able to organize and synthesize a chorus of voices from his past, with ongoing impressions, into musical form. I wondered if James could work with a therapist to strategize how to make this manner of managing voices more conscious. A musician performer can act as a "meta-communicator" (Mindell, 1988) or an observing ego, which a patient still in the wake of a mental health crisis may lack. That meta-communicator—which may be Eminem, or Leonard Cohen—can structure and express emotional material and experiences until the patient arrives home again (Berlyne, 1971; Mindell, 1988).

Another way in which listening with patients to music was useful in individual and group sessions was when fragments of patients' identities were split off and held in pieces of music. Seneca's feelings about betrayal and abandonment by his mother were exalted in Eminem's "Cleaning Out My Closet" (Eminem & Bass, 2002, Track 4). Traumatized aspects of a younger self could also be split off and held in various pieces of music like "somatic markers" (Damasio, 1995), such as when Manu projected his split-off Pacific

Island childhood into the music of IZ. Initially, Manu rejected IZ's music and then later revisited it in a sentimental manner. Another patient asked to revisit James Taylor and Carole King's duet of, "You can Close Your Eyes" (Taylor, 1971/2010, Track 15) while working through deferred grief about the loss of her marriage. She learned to tolerate the song for longer periods of time as she worked through loss. Another patient explored her attachment to the song "Spirit in the Sky" (Greenbaum, 1969, Track 1) as a way to face a foreclosed, traumatized aspect of her self (Ready, 2013).

Many of the patients described in these chapters preferred music that induced negative emotions (i.e., sadness, anger). Martindale and Moore (1988) proposed that listeners are suspended, when listening to negative emotional music, in a disassociated state wherein there is neural activation that produces enjoyment as long as the person remains within a safe aesthetic environment. Schubert (2010) elaborated on the dissociative state as "transportative," and emphasized the importance of the protected environment in which music was experienced. This element of perceived "safety" becomes more delicate when working with patients who have trauma histories. Having a clinician in the room when listening to emotionally provocative music may help maintain an environment of safety for a patient. This was the case for both Hannah and Harika, who were able to process sorrow with music resonating in the background.

Music can help create a therapeutic frame and maintain the co-created safe space of a group or dyad within which patients can express, and learn to abide, such emotions as frustration, anger, depression, grief, and desolation. When music incites strong affect in patients, a clinician can help individual group members metabolize emotions together. Using music to engage with patients who are experiencing intense, acute depression or refractory depression can be a very gradual process. Jane, for example, protested that she had formerly loved music. In fact she had been a dancer, but she had become adverse to music—wanting to shut down or short circuit any song she heard playing, even in her church. It took several months for Jane to build up tolerance for her favorite Mary J. Blige CD, which she eventually brought to share with others in treatment.

When using music as an adjunct tool with patients who are experiencing severe mental health disturbances, it's important to keep in mind that music can sometimes stimulate negative associations, emotional anguish, or unbearable pleasant or ambivalent feelings in patients. In the worst-case scenario, music could exacerbate psychosis. In many cases, psychosis can serve as a defense against the pleasures and pains of daily life. Because the patient has not experienced positive, corrective use of projective identification by a primary caregiver who could not—or would not—metabolize her child's raw emotions, the psychotic person may attack the building blocks of thoughts and feelings and any internal or external attempts at linking (Bion, 1959/1984a, 1962; Symington & Symington, 1996). In a sense, the psychotic person's senses act in reverse operation, as hallucinosis (Bion, 1965). Rather than taking in sensations, the patient may push them back out into the environment, and attach undesirable, negative feelings to them.

On the most acute hospital units I set a concrete frame, using a white board to convey basic ground rules of time, space, and expectations around tolerance. Patients were asked to listen without comment while a song played. Open discussion and song requests occurred between songs. Each patient's responses were written verbatim on the white board. Responses could be associative, non-linear, or even tangentially pertinent to the song. Patients were encouraged to speak out if a song were too agitating or otherwise intolerable, in which case we would stop the offending song. Other protocols included keeping the iPod and portable speaker in the same location and having only one person in charge of monitoring the device.

The most challenging groups occurred when I failed to set or uphold a strong frame. One of my first attempts at using music with acute psychiatric patients was in a poorly framed group on the subject of grief. Several patients who had just arrived at the hospital were escorted into the group. I established vague ground rules. After fumbling with the electronic equipment, I launched without sufficient introduction into Mozart's "Requiem" (1791, Track 1). One of the new patients became restless. She looked anxiously down her aisle and around the room for an escape. She stood up and abruptly announced, "I need to go. Now. Now!" A staff member accompanied her back to the acute unit where, I later learned, she devolved into a full-blown psychotic episode. The experience taught me to be cautious and to move slowly in case music engaged unanticipated memories and unconscious responses (Konecni, 2008).

Sometimes, the mere rhythmic appeal of a piece of music was a strong connecting force. Among patients experiencing psychosis, there was a near universal draw to the music of Michael Jackson. He seemed to be the master of inspiring listeners to tap into their own ability to sense a regular pulse in an auditory signal as another form of touch. A steady beat, such as with "Billie Jean" or "Human Nature," seemed to help individuals synchronize together in movement (Honing, 2002; Lerdahl & Jackendoff, 1983; Winkler et al., 2009). In terms of classical music, various renditions of Baroque Adagios seemed consistently relaxing and organizing for patients, as if the music spoke directly to the parasympathetic nervous system, inducing a sense of calm and balance (Miluk-Kolasa, Matejek, & Stupnicki, 1996).

Working with Anna (chapter 5), I first learned how music could help establish a co-created setting in which trauma could be expressed and processed through performance in a dyad. Next I would like to explore a performance-based reconstruction process in a group setting. Mike, an Iraq veteran, performed the steps of a traumatic memory while participating in a group. With music as a mediating force he gradually altered his intense emotional responses. Mike had experienced the death of several young soldiers under his command. Full of rage when he arrived on the acute unit, Mike spit at staff and threatened other patients. He seemed to be re-living Iraq battles, which he projected on to hospital hallways. He reluctantly participated in groups. First he leaned against the far wall of the room listening to songs. Then he began executing dance steps in a square formation on the sidelines. Mike eventually migrated his dances to the front of the room. He would gesture as if he were handing out food rations to fellow soldiers.

As Mike participated more in groups, he began speaking openly with staff and peers about war memories. His stories were mainly focused on the battalion of young soldiers in his charge. Two soldiers had saved Mike's life—and sacrificed their own—while all of them were in captivity. Mike expressed guilt and gratitude. He repeated the story leading up to the soldiers' deaths in the same careful manner he performed the dance steps, every afternoon for two weeks. He encouraged other patients to join him in dancing. Then he would stop and flail, arms spinning, as if desperately trying to brace against a fall. The rhythm of the two sections of his dance seemed to parallel his internal processes of shame, forgiveness, and redemption.

For his final few days of performances Mike selected the Jackson Five's "Dancing Machine" (David, Fletcher, & Parks, 1974, Track 17). He performed the square steps and the flailing dance, pleased when other patients danced beside him, mirroring his steps. By the time Mike discharged from the hospital, he spoke coherently and directly about his war experiences, including guilt and ambivalence about surviving when other soldiers died. Mike's ability to discuss the source of his agony might have been facilitated by having young male patients dancing with him. It may have also been symbolically important that he was safely contained while he reconstructed his war narrative. In any case, music was the medium through which, and within which, Mike refashioned painful memories.

We have seen how music has the power to transform therapeutic spaces and to incite both pleasant and traumatic implicit memories for the purpose of clinical work. For Anna, music transformed a small, empty room into a nightclub. A Mendelssohn piano piece stimulated and soothed Harika's unresolved grief.

Sharing a patient's musical world may be an entry into the antechamber of the unconscious, which may be an ideal place to allow space for co-created dialogue. Matt's comfort with moving between dissociation and presence was communicated through song choices. In selecting Vega songs, Matt could convey a sense of longing for the attention of an aloof mother, while expressing his preference for cool detachment. Matt's songs provided clues on how to rhythmically attune to him (Beebe & Stern, 1977; Knoblaugh, 2005).

With patients diagnosed with borderline personality disorder establishing rapport—with or without music—was often a shared walk through a labyrinth. Randi was a thirty-five-year-old patient who had a history of childhood trauma, including sexual abuse by relatives. In the hospital, she would engage in intense re-enactments that included hiding under furniture and banging her head against the walls. Music and drawing were two activities Randi identified as calming, although music without words was intensely agitating for her. She found Cash's "Folsom Prison Blues" (Cash & Jenkins, 1968) comforting, and Leonard Cohen's "Suzanne" (Cohen, 1967). Yo-Yo Ma playing Bach would send her yowling, wrapped in a blanket, under a desk. In individual sessions, Randi wanted to listen to her favorite music while discussing the clinical aspects of using music. She preferred to role-play that she was the clinician and I was her patient. Building rapport with Randi involved allowing her to have agency in deciding the direction of the session. She gradually introduced small bits of classical music into her playlist. In the process of learning to tolerate, and articulate her emotional responses, Randi gradually began using music (including classical) to help broaden her thinking about her next steps in recovery.

A music listening device used in conjunction with therapy can be particularly beneficial in helping BPD patients and those with PTSD in the process of reality testing and managing trauma-related anxiety (Decety & Chaminade, 2005; Hug & Lohne, 2009; Ruby & Decety, 2001). Because music facilitates an enhanced non-verbal connection (Rubin & Niemeier, 1992; Schore, 2001), it is a powerful modality in helping to bypass defenses and denial in working with such patients (Hug & Lohne, 2009; Olivier, 2006).

One example of using music in this manner centered around Janice, who had been struggling with command hallucinations and intense trauma responses to her surrounding environments since a motor vehicle accident at age 48 that resulted in physical injuries to her cervical vertebrae. The feelings of being out of control caused by the accident instigated the reemergence of memories involving abuse and sexual trauma from Janice's pre-teen years. By the time I started working with Janice, she was highly vigilant about anyone sitting close to her. She was easily unsettled by environmental stimuli that even tangentially referenced her trauma. The first time I noticed her reactivity was when I played an obscure Hank Williams song during a process group. Janice left the room; she was trembling. She said she was close to having a panic attack. Conversely, when I played Led Zeppelin or Journey, Janice became calmer.

I asked Janice if we could begin experimenting with using music as a tool for managing her voices and for the intrusion of traumatic memories. We chose one or two Hank Williams songs that reminded Janice of her abusive stepfather. Then we chose several "safe" songs such as Journey's "Don't Stop

Believin" (Cain, Perry, & Schon, 1981, Track 2) and Led Zeppelin's' "Going to California" (Page & Plant, 1971). Janice and I decided on the structure of the experiment together. First we established goals. She wanted to be able to attend groups and other social events. As it was, she was could only stay in the room if she sat in a particular chair, facing the door. If she sat on the couch she worried that someone aggressive would sit beside her. She also became notably flustered and even dissociative when trying to locate an open seat in a crowded room. Janice agreed to wear earphones while listening to her preferred music to create a sound buffer. Likewise, she could don the earphones if, when seated in a group, someone who frightened her sat beside her. Music helped create space. Janice was eventually able to sit through entire groups (and later films in public movie theaters) with less vigilance.

The second part of our experiment related to modulating emotions. First we chose an unsettling Hank Williams song. At first I regulated the volume or changed the song entirely according to Janice's commands. We would try to pinpoint at what moment in the song Janice noticed herself starting to dissociate. She would make an affirmative gesture or I would check with her if I noticed that she seemed distant and unfocused. Once Janice acknowledged that the song was disturbing, we would switch to one of her favorite songs until Janice could focus again. Janice could also request that I turn down the volume when she found a song disturbing. We would discuss at what volume the song became benign. Eventually Janice modulated and switched songs herself, and without prompting. These experiments were meant to provide Janice with a new context for working with trauma and emotions and to encourage her confidence.

Most recently, I have been experimenting with using patient-selected music for transitions in groups. I have also begun using music as a coping and sensitivity training technique for patients who hear voices—in coordination with materials from The Hearing Voices Network (2015) website—or who have identified high sensitivity to sound or sensory integration issues. Prior to the music listening activity, we discuss sound tolerance in terms of such elements as rhythm, volume, tone, presentation, lyrics, and authenticity of the singer's voice. We take turns alternately playing beloved pieces of music or irritating pieces of music. Anyone in the group is welcome to request volume change, or termination of the song. Whenever possible the person who halts or changes the song explains what stimulated their response before selecting the next song. The group has been particularly popular with young adults experiencing psychosis. It has offered a platform for intergenerational conversation and connection among otherwise socially isolated people.

Another area of clinical utility for music would be to adapt the progressive mirroring work of Benedetti and Peccecia (Koehler, 2006) in which patient and therapist sit back to back modifying one another's drawings. Exchanging turns in song choices, modifying lyrics, or creating a dialogue consisting of each person's beloved musical pieces are possibilities with individuals. These methods would allow patients to integrate divergent aspects of self: a longing to connect conflicting with an urge to reject connection and return to an isolated state.

Over time, in using music with individuals and with groups, I noticed themes emerge of shared musical values among patients. There was a common concern with familiarity, perception of melody, a steady rhythm (although the intensity and layers of rhythm varied), and the quality, tone, and authenticity (i.e., lived experience) of a singer's voice. Patients also preferred music that matched their emotional state. Elliot requested and rejected songs depending on a fluctuating mood. These concerns for familiarity and for the music to match a listener's emotion aligned with contemporary research evidence (Hargreaves & North, 1995; Sluckin, Hargreaves, & Colmman, 1982; Evans & Schubert, 2008).

I have found no consistent correlation between diagnoses and musical preference other than anecdotally. A number of studies have attempted to draw correlations between young people's musical preferences and various personality disordered traits (Forsyth, Barnard, & McKegany, 1997), looking for early indicators of mental illness. Other inquiries have explored "whether music can instigate drug use violence, suicide and antisocial behavior" (Baker & Bor, 2008, p. 285). It seems prudent and humane to regard music preference on a case-by-case basis. I'm concerned that faulty deductions that could easily be made about young people's musical preferences being pathological (Ballard & Coates, 1995). For example, if a high incidence of young adults with heavy metal music preferences are hospitalized for psychiatric problems (Rosenbaum & Prinsky, 1991), this does not prove that listening to heavy metal music is an early indicator of a psychiatric problem.

The results of music/behavioral correlation studies are mixed and sometimes contradictory. As an example, preferences for heavy metal music have been linked with assertiveness, aggressiveness, moodiness, pessimism, discontent, and impulsiveness (Wells & Hakanen, 1991). A Canadian study (Lacourse, Claes, & Veleneuve, 2001) showed the opposite results—that heavy metal music preferences were associated with positive changes in affect. Popular music as a preference has been linked with values such as being overly responsible, role-conscious, involved in struggles with sexual identity issues, seeking acceptance, and seeking to find a balance between dependence and independence (Wells & Hakanen, 1991).

Chapter 9

Conclusion

While in the process of writing this book, I was diagnosed with an aggressive advanced breast cancer. I listened to Beethoven's "Fidelio" (1805), and Nick Drake for hours during chemotherapy treatment. The music sifted and ordered layers of complex emotions, providing comfort while it structured, symbolized, and carried an emotionally precarious experience. A dosage machine delivering chemotherapy drugs clicked in counterpoint rhythm. Listening to music during treatments made it easier to remain in a calm and receptive state. Otherwise, it seemed counterintuitive to welcome toxic cancer–killing chemicals that simultaneously and paradoxically killed healthy cells.

The experience of being tagged with a chronic, allegedly incurable, illness stimulated feelings of uncertainty, powerlessness, and fear. These unsettling affects were soothed and scaffolded equally, albeit differently, by Bach passion masses, and Van Morrison blues ballads. Undergoing chemotherapy, mediated by music, helped facilitate new insight into what it must be like for a person caught up in the psychological and physiological chaos of a severe chronic mental health condition. I imagine that person would undergo even stronger waves of confounding emotions that surge and ebb and sometimes storm. When riding such waves in seas of passionate uncertainty, a patient might find that the music of Aerosmith or Poison might better apprehend crashing feelings that possess, as Stern (1985) observed, musical dimensions of duration, frequency, and intensity. When we are in raw and vulnerable human states, music may hold more resonance for us than language.

There is an abundance of ways in which music can be a useful tool for clinicians, even if a clinician never invites music into the therapeutic session. Music may be part of the clinician's own metabolization or reverie process. A therapist might sit in his empty office writing session notes while listening to Miles Davis or Bob Dylan. He may practice a Beethoven sonata on his piano or an Eric Clapton guitar riff to transition at home after a long day of appointments. Listening to beloved music—by that I mean paying close attention to notes and nuances, and allowing his observing ego to follow an emotional narrative, while noticing emerging patterns, ideas, and interpretations—might be one essential part of a sustainable clinical practice. Perhaps listening to music could be akin for clinicians to practicing scales as a way of becoming attuned to the vicissitudes of life.

Another way to employ music in a therapeutic practice involves clinicians using music indirectly as part of establishing a safe and aesthetic frame in the service of encouraging attunement and trust with hard-to-reach patients. Music, used in this manner, may expand a clinician's capacity through heightened awareness of sense and sound to attune to a patient's preferred rhythm, cadence, pitch, volume, and tone. It may also allow a therapist to be more embodied in his moment-to-moment awareness of emotional shifts occurring in the therapeutic dyad (Bion, 1984; Knobluach, 2000; 2005). A therapist could choose, for example, to match, or counterbalance, the rapid pace of a patient rapping a manic banter of details. A therapist could introduce dissonance, or clap hands, to jar a monotonous exchange marked by flat affect.

Another benefit of including patient's music in clinical sessions is that self-selected music can help shift unequal power dynamics between clinician and patient that might otherwise stimulate caution or paranoia. Patients are experts on their own musical preferences. They may need help integrating their unconscious understanding of music's emotional impact into conscious awareness. If we always preference our own aesthetic, including musical, taste we limit the potential for an embodied connection.

A clinician chooses baroque music for her waiting room because it has a calming effect for her. The same music sends a patient into a cold sweat due to his memories of a critical mother who directed the high school orchestra. To mediate his anxiety the patient arrives for the next session wearing earphones hooked to a personal listening device. The patient listens to Pink, or Pink Floyd, or Public Enemy. What would happen if the clinician merely inquired about the patient's music choice, thus inviting it by proxy into the room? Let us imagine that we are discussing a teenage or a young adult female patient who professes to love Beyoncé, whom she calls "Queen B." What would the clinician learn if he streamed Beyoncé-style songs on Pandora while reflecting on the young woman's fledgling sense of identity? By the term "listening," I mean to concentrate in an active manner suggested by Keats' (1817) in the term "negative capability." The term was later adapted by Bion (1984) to mean being present without grasping after memory or desire. Music can be an especially effective adjunct tool with patients who are already able to use music as a primary form of self-expression and self-organization. What becomes more challenging for a clinician is—as I noted when first listening to Tool with several patients—when he finds the patient's music offensive, insipid, or unattractive.

My opera-loving uncle once stored my young adult record collection for one year while I lived in Japan. Upon my return he told me that my musical tastes were "pedestrian, peripheral, shallow, and cloying." My collection included rock, folk, bluegrass, jazz, experimental jazz, and popular classical collections. He gave me a hand-drawn musical pyramid. At the erudite pinnacle he had placed Wagner, directly below he had located Beethoven, and Mozart. At the base of the pyramid was Bach. "Memorize this," he said. I wonder, in retrospective fantasy, what might have opened between my uncle and myself, if my eclectic musical taste had been allowed equal status and consideration in his music parlor. Although we can agree that musical forms have varying degrees of complexity and sophistication, there is no empirical proof that the degree of musical complexity equals greater potential for attunement or for building initial rapport with the majority of patients. Perhaps both the clinician and the patient would have the opportunity to become more appreciative of, or at least able to tolerate, one another's musical taste over time.

As I mentioned in the first chapter of this book, I began employing music with patients under the inherited assumption that classical music followed by classical jazz would be the penultimate genres for facilitating depth work. Now I believe, especially since proof is emerging that popular and non-classical music may be more effective in reducing symptoms of psychosis, that it is best to begin with a patient's beloved music. Inviting patient's preferred music into the therapeutic potential space, and working directly by listening to music together in either an individual or a group session, may seem radical, unbounded, or unwise to more seasoned clinicians. For one thing, a shared listening experience has the possibility of disrupting or destabilizing the frame and the balance of the dyad. Shared music may also introduce a level of intimacy and parity that is initially uncomfortable for both parties. Because music can incite physiological as well as emotional responses in patients and therapists, allowing music into the clinical hour also requires clinicians to contend with the body, or allowing embodiment as an element of the therapeutic connection what Aron and Anderson (1998) referred to as "a jointly created skin-ego/breathing self" (p. 25). Music can "touch" both patient and therapist by inciting emotions and such physiological (and possibly countertransference) responses as chills, anxiety, or repulsion. Music would also open other avenues for potential—and perhaps less threatening—interpretations of unconscious material the music would offer to both parties.

The strongest, most expedient clinical links I have been able to establish with patients occurred while attuning and mis-attuning to their preferred songs. Once a connection was established with a patient, music could be used to help with social anxiety, paranoia, or trauma responses while gradually introducing new forms of music and working with metaphor, sound, and symbol toward reintegration. My fantasy is that we could learn to incorporate personal music devices as inexpensive interpersonal mediators, affect modulators, and environmental enhancers. Music devices serve as objects of self-representation, integration, and transition.

One more caveat: I do not mean to imply that music makes working with hard-to-reach patients an easier prospect. Eigen (1993) referred to therapy with psychosis as a "messy and harrowing business" (p. 18). I noticed that while digesting these case studies, before compiling them into written narratives, I felt a magnified presence of abiding primal fears, such as fears of annihilation, abandonment, and betrayal. My countertransference sent me searching restlessly and relentlessly through online journals for true crime, and natural catastrophes, in proportion to the degree of silence and transference within a particular patient's story. What initially seemed to be a superficial and uneventful session later turned out to be exhausting to capture in words. It was more difficult to contain and metabolize music that I found unfamiliar, or displeasing.

For patients undergoing the stress and trauma of hospitalization, access to music devices both individually and as a tool of collective engagement is essential. Music can provide forums for patients to share their inner worlds with clinicians and with family members. Even the simple act of inviting (or downloading) a patient's preferred music can inspire communication.

As illustrated in the cases of Harika and Manu, clinicians could explore using music as an adjunct therapeutic tool with patients from other cultures for whom English is neither the predominant language, nor the language of early implicit experience. Music may be more culturally familiar in terms of melody, and voice, than language translations when a patient is suffering. Listening to music with a therapist helps regulate intensified feelings of alienation.

My deepest wish in writing this book is to encourage exploration of the clinical uses of music as an adjunct therapeutic tool in attuning with difficult-to-reach patients. Music can be especially effective with young adults who can become frozen in normal developmental tasks. If young people are attached to their personal music devices as extensions of themselves, then we as clinicians can join with them in their musical worlds to help them reintegrate toward self-determination in a respectful, sensitive, and non-stigmatizing manner.

I will close this book, in the manner in which it opened, with a musical scene—a transcendent moment to which words would have added nothing. At seventy-three, my beloved uncle began experiencing dementia, which impacted his capacity to paint. One day, after his verbal and artistic abilities had all but abandoned him, we sat listening to music in his parlor. He had a full-time nurse by then. The light was falling toward evening. I put on the overture from "Tristan and Isolde" with Jessye Norman singing the part of Isolde. The overture filled the room with its unresolved longing. My uncle was in a wheelchair. I was in an overstuffed chair. We sat knee to knee, quietly listening to the scratchy record. The music expressed both yearning for boundless love and dread for its imminent loss. We were preparing for a mutual surrender. His mind was unraveling; my mind was trying to wrap at once around presence and annihilation. We shared a profound, connected moment before he retreated into complete silence, into primal space, a transcendence, and absence from his own body, and from his beloved crimson and gold parlor. Dust swirled in the air. Night pressed at windows. By the time the song ended, both of us were in tears. The music had articulated and created a space, or portal, wherein our implicit selves met and parted.

Bibliography

A[...] usic and altered states: Consciousness, tran[...] London, UK: Jessica Kingsley.
[...] müklü, M., & Akvardar, Y. (2009). Prevalence [...] oms: In the city of Izmir, Turkey. *Social Psy-[...]y, 44*(11), 905–910.
[...] New York, NY: W.W. Norton & Company.
[...] 2004). *Practice guideline for the treatment of* [...] ington, DC: Author.
[...] anguage, and communication disorders: I. Clini-[...], evaluation of their reliability. *Archives of Gen-*

[...] J. (2008). My way. [Recorded by F. Sinatra] On [...] wnload]. New York, NY: Reprise.
[...] ger, L., Perto, G., & Munk-Jørgensen, P. (2005). [...] d subsequent schizophrenia-spectrum disorders: [...] nt cases. *British Journal of Psychiatry, 187*(6), [...].510.

[...], 39). Somewhere over the rainbow. [Recorded by I. Kamakawiwo'ole & J. D. Mello, Conductor] On *Facing future* [CD]. Honolulu, HI: Mountain Apple. (1987)

Arnett, J. (1995). Adolescents' uses of the media for self-socialization. *Journal of Youth and Adolescence, 24*(5), 519–533. doi:10.1007/BF01537054.

Aron, L. & Anderson, F. S. (1998). *Relational perspectives on the body.* New York: Routledge Press.

Bach, J. S. (1713–1714). Concerto in D minor No. 3 after Alessandro Marcello. [Recorded by G. Gould, Performer] On *Glenn Gould and serenity* [CD]. New York, NY: Sony Classical. (2003)

Bach, J. S. (1717–1723) Air on a G string: Orchestral suite no. 3 in D major. [Recorded by T. Dart & N. Mariner, Conductor]. On *Baroque adagios* [CD]. New York, NY: Universal Music. (2002)

Bach, J. S. (1717–1723). Suite for solo cello no. 6 in D major. [Recorded by Yo-Yo-Ma]. On *Bach: The cello suites* [Digital download]. New York, NY: Sony BMG. (1997)

Bach, J. S. (1741). Variation 12: Canone al quarta. [Recorded by G. Gould]. On *Goldberg variations* [CD]. Toronto: Sony/BMG. (1956/2003).

Bach, J. S. (1741). A state of wonder. [Recorded by G. Gould] On *The complete Goldberg variations 1955 & 1981* [CD]. New York, NY: Sony/BMG Musical Entertainment. (1955/1981)

Bach, J. S., & Gounod, C. (1859). Ave Maria. [Recorded by S. Brightman]. On *Classics* [CD]. New York: NY. Studios. (2001)

Baker, F., & Bor, W. (2008). Can music preference indicate mental health status in young people? *Australasian Psychiatry, 16*(4), 284–288. doi:10.1080/10398560701879589.

Baldwin, J. (1998). Freaks and the American ideal of manhood. *James Baldwin: Collected Essays*, 814–29. New York: Penguin Books.

Barale, F. & Minazzi, V. (2008, October). Off the beaten track: Freud, sound and music. Statement of a problem and some historico-critical notes. *International Journal of Pscyhoanalysis, 89*(5), 937–57.

Beebe, B. (2003). Brief mother–infant treatment: Psychoanalytically informed video feedback. *Infant Mental Health Journal, 24*(1), 24–52.

Beebe, B. (2006). Co-constructing mother–infant distress in face-to-face interactions: Contributions of microanalysis. *Infant Observation, 9*(2), 151–164.

Beebe, B., & Lachmann, F. M. (1994). Representation and internalization in infancy: Three principles of salience. *Psychoanalytic Psychology, 11*(2), 127.

Beebe, B., & Stern, D. N. (1977). Engagement-disengagement and early object experiences. In N. Freedman & S. Grand (Eds.), *Communicative structures and psychic structures: A psychoanalytic interpretation of communication* (pp. 35–55). New York: Plenum Press.

Beethoven, L. V. (1796–1797). Piano concerto no. 1 in C major (Op. 15): Largo. [Recorded by L. O. Players & R. Norrington]. On *Beethoven: 5 piano concertos* [CD]. London, UK: EMI. (2008)

Beethoven, L. V. (1805). Fidelio [Recorded by K. Bohm and Staatskapelle Dresden]. On *Fidelio* [CD]. GmbH, Hamburg: Deutsch Grammophone. (2005)

Beethoven, L. V. (1819–1823). Missa solemnis in D major [Recorded by the Orchestre des Champs Elysees & P. Herrewegthe]. On *Missa solemni* [CD]. Paris, FR: Harmona Mundi. (1995)

Benjamin, J. (1998). *Like subjects, love objects: Essays on recognition and sexual difference*. New Haven, CT: Yale University Press.

Bentall, R. P. (2009). *Doctoring the mind: Why psychiatric treatments fail*. London: Penguin Books.

Berlyne, D. E. (1971). *Aesthetics and psychobiology*. NY, NY: Appleton-Century-Crofts.

Berry, J. W., Kim, U., Minde, T., & Mok, D. (1987). Comparative studies of acculturative stress. *International Migration Review, 21*, 490–511.

Binelli, M. (2008). The future according to Radiohead. *Rolling Stone, 1045*, 54–59. Retrieved from http://markbinelli.com.

Bion, W. R. (1959). Attacks on linking. *International Journal of Psychoanalysis*, 40, pp. 308–315.
———. (1962). A theory of thinking. In W. R. Bion, *Second thoughts: Selected papers on psychoanalysis (*pp. 110–119). London, UK: Heinemann.
———. (1963). *Elements of psycho-analysis*. London, UK: Karnac.
———. (1965). *Transformations*. London, UK: Heinemann.
———. (1984a). *Second thoughts: Selected papers on psychoanalysis*. New York, NY: Karnac.
———. (1984b). *Learning from experience*. London, UK: Karnac.
———. (1990). *Brazilian lectures*. New York: Karnac.
———. (1992). *Cogitations*. London, UK: Karnac. (Original work published in 1957).
Birchwood, M., Iqbal, Z., Chadwick, P., & Trower, P. (2000). Cognitive approach to depression and suicidal thinking in psychosis. 1. Ontogeny of post-psychotic depression. *British Journal of Psychiatry*, *177*, 516–521. doi:10.1192/bjp.177.6.516.
Bleandonu, G. (1994). *Wilfred Bion: His life and works 1897–1979*. New York, NY: Other Press.
Blos, P. (1962). *On adolescence. A psychoanalytic interpretation*. New York: The Free Press.
Bodle, A. (2014, September 11). Phil Collins saved me from suicide: the music that changed my life. *The Guardian*. Retrieved from http://theguardian.com.
Boke, O., Aker, S., Alptekin, A., Sarisoy, G., & Sahin, A. (2007). Schizophrenia in Turkish newspapers. *Social Psychiatry & Psychiatric Epidemiology*, *42*(6), 457–461. doi:10.1007/s00127-007-0198-8.
Bosnak, R. (2007). *Embodiment: Creative imagination in medicine, art, and travel*. London, UK: Routledge.
Bowman, D. (2010, January 30). Neighborhood girl. *The New York Times*. Retrieved from http://www.nytimes.com.
Brahms, J. (1859). Intermezzo no. 2 for piano in B-flat minor. [Recorded by G. Gould]. On *Glenn Gould and serenity* [CD]. New York, NY: Sony Music. (2003)
Brandt, A., Gebrian, M., & Slevc, R. (2012, September). Music and early language acquisition. *Frontiers in Auditory Cognitive Neuroscience*. 2012 doi: 10.3389/fpsyg.2012.00327.
Bronfman, E. (2008). Radiohead. *Time*, *171(*19), 120. Retrieved from EBSCO*host*.
Brown, A. (2009, October 12). Jason Derulo will save your relationship. *The LA Times Music Blog*. Retrieved from http://latimesblogs.latimes.com/music_blog/2009.
———. (2010, March 1). Jason Derulo's self-titled debut. *The LA Times: Album Review*: Retrieved from http://latimesblogs.latimes.com/music_blog.
Bucci, W. (1985). Dual coding: A cognitive model for psychoanalytic research. *Journal of the American Psychoanalytic Association 33*: 571–607.
Bucci, W. (1997). *Psychoanalysis and cognitive science: A multiple code theory*. New York: Guilford.
Burns, J., Labbé, E., Williams, K., & McCall, J. (1999). Perceived and physiological indicators of relaxation: As different as Mozart and Alice in Chains. *Applied Psychophysiology & Biofeedback*, *24*(3), 197–202. Retrieved from EBSCO*host*.

Cain, J., Perry, S., & Schon, N. (1981). Don't Stop Believin.' [Recorded by Journey] On *Escape* [Digital download]. Berkeley, CA: Columbia.

Cantor-Graae, E. (2007). The contribution of social factors to the development of schizophrenia: a review of recent findings. *Canadian Journal of Psychiatry, 52*(5), 287–294. Retrieved from EBSCO*host*.

Caramanica, J. (2008, October 22). Eminem resurfaces in a new role, memoirist. *The New York Times*. Retrieved from http://nytimes.com.

Carter, D. M. (2009). Drop the world. [Recorded by Lil Wayne]. On *Rebirth* [Digital download]. New York, NY: Cash Money Records.

Cash, J., & Jenkins, G. (1968). Folsom prison blues. [Recorded by J. Cash]. On *Live at folsom prison* [Digital download]. Folsom, CA: Columbia.

Charles, M. (2002). *Patterns: Building blocks of experience*. Hillsdale, NJ: The Analytic Press.

Charles, M. (2012). Working with trauma: Lessons from Bion and Lacan. New York: Jason Aronson, Inc.

Cheshire, N. M. (1996). The empire of the ear: Freud's problem with music. *International Journal of Psych-Analysis, 77*: 1127–68.

Cohen, L. (1967). Suzanne. On *The best of Leonard Cohen* [CD]. New York, NY: Columbia. (1975)

Cohen, L. (1975). Various. On *The Best of Leonard Cohen* [CD]. New York, NY: Columbia.

Cohen, M., Solowij, N., & Carr, V. (2008). Cannabis, cannabinoids and schizophrenia: integration of the evidence. *Australian & New Zealand Journal of Psychiatry, 42*(5), 357–368. doi:10.1080/00048670801961156.

Conrad, J. (1902/1999). *Heart of darkness*. London, UK: Penguin Classic.

Cosoff, S. J., Julian, H., & Cosoff, S. J. (1998). The prevalence of comorbid anxiety in schizophrenia, schizoaffective disorder and bipolar disorder. *Australian & New Zealand Journal of Psychiatry, 32*(1), 67–72. doi:10.1046/j.1440-1614.1998.00374.x.

Cox, R. (1990). A history of music. *Journal of Aesthetics & Art Criticism, 48*(4), 395–409. Retrieved from EBSCO*host*.

Cozolino, L. (2002). *The neuroscience of psychotherapy: Building and rebuilding the human brain*. New York, NY: W. W. Norton.

Damasio, A. (1995). *Descartes' error: Emotion, reason, and the human brain*. New York, NY: Avon.

David, H., Fletcher, D., & Parks, D. (1974). Dancing Machine. [Performed by The Jackson 5]. On *Jackson 5: The ultimate collection* [Digital download]. Hillsville, West LA: Motown.

Davidson, L., Tondora, J., Lawless, M. S., O'Connell, M. J., & Rowe, M. (2009). *A practical guide to recovery-oriented practice. Tools for transforming mental health care*. New York, NY: Oxford University Press.

Davis, M. (1959). So What. On *Kind of blue*. [Digital Download]. New York, NY: Sony.

Davoine, F., & Gaudillière, J. M. (2004). *History beyond trauma*. (S. Fairfield, Trans.) New York, NY: Other Press.

Darwin, C. (1871). *The descent of man, and selection in relation to sex.* London, UK: John Murray.
Dawkins. (1976). *The selfish gene.* Oxford, UK: Oxford University Press.
Decety, J., & Chaminade, T. (2005). The neurology of imitation and intersubjectivity. In S. Hurley & N. Chater (Eds.), *Perspectives on imitation: From neuroscience to social science.* Cambridge, MA: MIT Press.
Dede, M. (2010). http://worldmusic.nationalgeographic.com/view/ page.basic/ genre/ content.genre/turkish_pop/en_US. Retrieved on December 28, 2012.
Derulo, J. (2010). Ridin' solo. On *Jason Derulo* [Digital download]. New York, NY: Belugia Heights.
Dickerson, F. B. (2000). Cognitive behavioral psychotherapy for schizophrenia: A review of recent empirical studies. *Schizophrenia Research, 43*(2–3), 71–90. doi:10.1016/S0920-9964(99)00153-X.
Dieckmann, H. (1974). The constellation of the countertransference. In G. Adler (Ed.), *Success and failure in analysis.* New York, NY: Putnam.
Dissanayake, E. (2000). Antecedents of the temporal arts in early mother-infant interaction. In N.L. Wallin, B. Merker, & S. Brown (Eds.), *The origins of music,* 389–410. Cambrridge, MA: MIT Books.
Dissanayake, E. (2009). Root, leaf, blossom, or bole: Concerning the origin and adaptive function of music. In S. Malloch & S. Trevarthen (Eds.), *Communicative musicality: Exploring the basis of human companionship,* 17–30. New York: Oxford University Press.
Durkheim, E. (2006). *On suicide.* New York, NY: Penguin Books (Originally published in 1898).
Edna, G. (2008, June 30). Portishead sheds labels for 'third' round. *USA Today.* Retrieved from Academic Search Premier database.
Ehrzenweig, A (1975). *The psychoanalysis of artistic vision ad hearing.* (Third Edition). London: Shelton Press.
Eigen, M. (1993). *The psychotic core.* Northvale, NJ: Jason Aronson, Inc.
Ekman, P. (1992). An argument for basic emotions. *Cognition and emotion, 6,* 169–200.
Eligon, D. (2010, Mar 9). For Lil Wayne sentencing date yields a year at Rikers. *The New York Times.* Retrieved from http://nytimes.com.
Ellis, D. (1995). Dummy. *People, 43*(2), 27. Retrieved from Academic Search Premier database.
Emde, R. E. (1988). Development terminable & interminable II: Recent psychoanalytic theory and therapeutic considerations. *International Journal of Psych-Analysis, 69,* 283–296. Retrieved from EBSCO*host.*
Eminem & Bass, J. (2002). Cleanin out my closet. [Recorded by Eminem]. On *The Eminem show* [CD]. Los Angeles, CA: Shady Records.
Evans, P., & Schubert, E. (2008). Relationships between expressed and felt emotions in music. *Musicae Scientiae, 12*(1), 75–99. Retrieved from EBSCO*host.*
Eriksen, M., Hermandsen, T. E., Ghost, A., Dench, I., & Knowles, B. (2007). Beautiful liar. [Recorded by Beyoncé and Shakira] On *Beautiful liar* [Digital download]. NY, NY: Columbia.

Fachner, J. (2010). *Music therapy and addictions*. London, GBR: Jessica Kingsley.

Fairbairn, W.R.D. (1952). The repression and return of bad objects (with special references to the "war neuroses"). In *Psychoanalytic studies of the personality* (pp.59–81). London: Routledge & Kegan Paul

Feder, S. (1990).The nostalgia of Charles Ives: An essay in affects and music. In S. Feder, R. L. Karmel, and G. H. Pollock (Eds.), Psychoanalytic explorations in music (pp. 233–66). Madison, CT: International Universities Press.

Feder, S. (1993). Promissory notes: Method in music and applied psychoanalysis. In S. Feder, F. L. Karmel, and G. H. Pollock (Eds.), Psychoanalytic explorations in music. (pp. 3–19). Madison, CT: International Universities Press.

Feder, S. (2004, January). Music as simulacrum of mental life. Presented at *American Psychoanalytic Association,* New York. Retrieved from http://internationalpsycho-analysis.net/wp-content/uploads/2007/05/htm

Feinsilver, D. B. (1986). Pao's telescopic overview of treatment. In D. B. Feinsilver (Ed.), *Towards a comprehensive model for Schizophrenic Disorders*. Hillsdale, NJ: Analytic Press.

Ferenczi, S. (1929). The unwelcome child and his death-instinct. *International Journal of Psychoanalysis, 10,* 125–129.

Ficino, M. (1980). *The book of life*. (C. Boer Trans.) Dallas, Texas: Spring.

Fledderus, M., Bohlmeijer, E. T., Smit, F., & Westerhof, G. J. (2010). Mental health promotion as a new goal in public mental health care: A randomized controlled trial of an intervention enhancing psychological flexibility. *American Journal of Public Health, 100,* 2372–2378. doi:10.2105/AJPH.2010.196196

Forsey, K. (1985). Various. On *The Breakfast Club Soundtrack*. [Digital Download]. Los Angeles, CA: A & M.

Freeman, D. (1998). *The fateful hoaxing of Margaret Mead: A historical analysis of her Samoan research*. Boulder, CO: Westview.

Frere-Jones, S. (2008). Spooky perfection. *The New Yorker, 84*(10), 138–139. Retrieved from Academic Search Premier database.

Freud, S. (1953). The Moses of Michelangelo. In J. Strachey (Ed. & Trans.), *The standard edition of the complete psychological works of Sigmund Freud* (Vol. 13. pp. 211–36). London, UK: Hogarth Press. (Original work published 1914)

Freud, S. (1957). The future prospects of psycho-analytic therapy. In J. Strachey (Ed. & Trans.), *The standard edition of the complete psychological works of Sigmund Freud* (Vol. 11. pp. 139–215). London, UK: Hogarth Press. (Original work published 1910)

Freud, S. (1964). New introductory lectures on psycho-analysis. In J. Strachey (Ed. & Trans.), *The standard edition of the complete psychological works of Sigmund Freud* (Vol. 18, pp. 1–182). London, UK: Hogarth Press. (Original work published 1933)

Fromm, E. (1965). Hyponanalysis: Theor and two case excerpts. *Psychotherapy: Theory, Research and Practice, 2*:127–133.

Fromm-Reichmann, F. (1959). *Psychoanalysis and psychotherapy*. Chicago, IL: University of Chicago Press. (Original work published 1946)

Frizzelle, C. (2012, August 12). The woman in 606. *The Stranger*. Retrieved from www.thestranger.com

Garfield, D. (2001). Chapter 10: The use of vitality affects in the coalescence of self in psychosis. *Progress in Self Psychology, 17,* 113–128. Retrieved from PEP Archive database

Gershwin, I. & Gershwin, G. (1926). Someone to Watch Over Me. [Recorded by C. Baker]. On *My Funny Valentine* [Digital download]. NY, NY: Blue Note (1953).

Gibbons, B. (1994a). It could be sweet. [Recorded by Portishead]. On *Dummy* [Digital download]. London, UK: Got Disc.

Gibbons, B. (1994b). Mysteron. [Recorded by Portishead]. On *Dummy* [Digital download]. London, UK: Got Disc.

Gibbons, B. (1994c). Numb. [Recorded by Portishead]. On *Dummy* [Digital download]. London, UK: Got Disc.

Gillespie, D. (1942). Night in Tunisia. [Recorded by B. Powell]. On *Blue Note Café Paris* [Digital download]. Paris, FR: EPS (1961)

Giroud, C., Felber, F., Augsburger, M., Horisberger, L., Rivier, L. & Mangin, P. (2000). Salvia divinorum: An hallucinogenic mint which might become a new recreational drug in Switzerland. *Forensic Science International, 112*(2) 143–150.

Glickson, J. & Cohen, Y. (2000). Can music alleviate cognitive dysfunction in schizophrenia? *Psychopathology, 33,* 43–47.

Gluck, M. T. (1762). Dance of the blessed spirits. [Recorded by M. T. Garatti & N. Mariner]. On *Baroque adagios* [CD]. Various: Decca. (2002)

Gold, C., Solli, H. P., Krüger, V., & Lie, S. A. (2009). Dose–response relationship in music therapy for people with serious mental disorders: Systematic review and meta-analysis. *Clinical Psychology Review, 29*(3), 193–207. doi:10.1016/j.cpr.2009.01.001.

Goldman, J. J. (1995). Vole. [Recorded by D. Dion]. On *D'eux* [Digital download]. Paris, France: Columbia.

Gordon, D. (2003). We regret to inform you that Radiohead still sounds weird. *Newsweek, 141*(23), 58. Retrieved from EBSCO*host.*

Gould, G. (2003). Various. On *Glenn Gould and serenity [CD].* New York: Sony Classical.

Graf, M. (1942). Reminiscences of Professor Sigmund Freud. *Psychoanalytic Quarterly, 11*: 465–76.

Green, A., Jordan, F., & Fairfax, Jr. R. (1977). Belle [Recorded by A. Green]. On *The Belle Album* [Digital Download]. Memphis: TN. Hi Records.

Greenbaum N. (1969). Spirit in the sky [Recorded by Norman Greenbaum] On *Spirit in the Sky.* [Digital download]. London, UK: Reprise Records.

Grotstein, J. (1977). The psychoanalytic concept of schizophrenia: I. The dilemma. *International Journal of Psycho-Analysis, 58,* 403–425. Retrieved from PEP Archive database.

Grotstein, J. S. (1981). *Splitting and projective identification.* Lanham, MD: Jason Aronson.

Grotstein, J. (1990). Nothingness, meaninglessness, chaos, and the "black hole" II— The black hole. *Contemporary Psychoanalysis, 26,* 377–407. Retrieved from PEP Archive database.

Grotstein, J. (1995a). Orphans of the "Real": I. Some modern and postmodern perspectives on the neurobiological and psychosocial dimensions of psychosis and other primitive mental disorders. *Bulletin of the Menninger Clinic, 59*(3), 287–311. Retrieved from Psychology and Behavioral Sciences Collection database.

Grotstein, J. (1995b). Orphans of the "Real": II. The future of object relations theory in the treatment of the. *Bulletin of the Menninger Clinic,* 59(3), 312–332. Retrieved from Psychology and Behavioral Sciences Collection database.

Grotstein, J. S. (2007). *A beam of intense darkness.* London, UK: Karnac.

Haasen, C., Yagdiran, O., Mass, R., & Krausz, M. (2000). Potential for misdiagnosis among Turkish migrants with psychotic disorders: A clinical controlled study in Germany. *Acta Psychiatrica Scandinavica, 101*(2), 125–129. doi:10.1034/j.1600-0447.2000.90065.x.

Hall, W. (1998). Cannabis use and psychosis. *Drug Alcohol Review, 17*(4), 433–444. doi:10.1080/09595239800187271.

Handel, F. (2002). Concerto grosso in A minor [Recorded by Academy of St. Martin in the Fields & N. Mariner]. On *Baroque adagios* [CD]. New York, NY: Universal Classical Group. (1739)

Hargreaves, D. J., & North, A. (1999). The functions of music in everyday life: Redefining the social in music psychology. *Psychology of Music, 27*(1), 71–83.

Harrer, G. & Harrer, H. (1977). Music, emotion, and autonomic function. In M. Critchley and R. A. Henson (Eds.), *Music and the brain.* London: Heinemann Medical Books.

Hearing Voices Network (2015). Retrieved at http://www.hearingvoicesusa.org/.

Henquet, C., Krabbendam, L., Spauwen, J., et al. (2005). Prospective cohort study of cannabis use predisposition for psychosis and psychotic symptoms in young people. *British Medical Journal, 330*(7481), 11–14. doi:10.1136/bmj.38267.664086.63.

Herrman, H., Saxena, S., & Moodie, R. (Eds.) (2005). *Promoting mental health: concepts, emerging evidence, practice* (A WHO Report in Collaboration with the Victorian Health Promotion Foundation and the University of Melbourne). Geneva: World Health Organization. Retrieved from http://who.int.

Hill, R. (1931, August). Mendelssohn as man and artist. *Gramophone.* Retrieved from http://www.gramophone.net.

Hogarty, G. E., Greenwald, D., Ulrich, R. F., Kornblith, S. J., DiBarry, A., Cooley, S., & Flesher, S. (1997). Three-year trials of personal therapy among schizophrenic patients living with or independent of family: II. Effects of adjustment of patients. *The American Journal of Psychiatry, 154*(11), 1514–1524. Retrieved from EBSCO*host.*

Holden, S. (2010, January 29). Still Cooly in control of her life and songs. *The New York Times.* Retrieved from http://www.nytimes.com.

Holmes, L. (1983). South Seas squall. *Sciences, 23*(4), 14. Retrieved from Academic Search Premier database.

Honing, H. (2002). Structure and interpretation of rhythm and timing. *Dutch Journal of Music Theory, 7,* 227–232.

Hooley, J. M., & Campbell, C. (2002). Control and controllability: Beliefs and behavior in high expressed emotion relatives. *Psychological Medicine: A Journal of Research in Psychiatry and the Allied Sciences, 32*(6), 1091–1099. doi:10.1017/S0033291702005779.

Hooley, J. M., & Gotlib, I. H. (2000). A diathesis-stress conceptualization of expressed emotion and clinical outcome. *Applied & Preventive Psychology, 9*(3), 135–151. doi:10.1016/S0962-1849(05)80001-0.

Hovey, J. D., & King, C. A. (1996). Acculturative stress, depression, and suicidal ideation among immigrant and second-generation Latino adolescents. *Journal of the American Academy of Child & Adolescent Psychiatry, 35*(9), 1183–1192. doi:10.1097/00004583-199609000-00016.

Howard, B. (1954). Fly me to the moon [Recorded by F. Sinatra, & C. B. Orchestra]. On *Down with love soundtrack* [Digital download]. Los Angeles, CA: Reprise Records (2003).

Howlett, L. (1997). Climbatize [Recorded by Prodigy]. On *The fat of the land* [Digital download]. London, UK: XL/Maverick.

Hug, E., & Lohne, P. (2009, February 1). A case study of the treatment of a patient with psychosis and drug dependence: Towards an integration of psychoanalytic and neuorscientific perspective. *Psychosis 1*(1), 82–92. Retrieved from EBSCO*host*.

Humphries, S. (2007, October 12). In rainbows. *The Christian Science Monitor, 9*(222), 13. Retrieved from EBSCO*host*.

Hurley, J., & Wilkins, R. (1968). Son of a preacher man [Recorded by D. Springfield]. On *Dusty in Memphis* [Digital download]. Memphis, TN: Atlantic.

Jackson, M. (1983). Beat It [Performed by M. Jackson]. On *Thriller* [Digital download]. Los Angeles, CA: EPIC.

Jackson, M. (1987). Bad [Performed by M. Jackson]. On *Bad* [Digital download]. Los Angeles, CA: EPIC.

Jagger, M., & Richards, K. (1973). Angie [Recorded by The Rolling Stones]. On *Goat's head soup* [Digital download]. Kingston, Jamaica: Universal International Music.

Jansson, P. & Fuemana, P. (1995). How Bizarre [Recorded by OMC]. On *How Bizarre.* [Digital download]. Auckland, NZ: huh! Records.

Joplin, S. (1902). The Entertainer [Recorded from piano roll by S. Joplin]. On *Scott Joplin: The Entertainer* [Digital download]. LA, CA: Shout Factory (2003).

Jung (1969). The psychological foundation of belief in spirits. In H. Read, M. Fordham, G. Adler, & W. McGuire (Eds.), *The collected works of C. G. Jung* (R. F. C. Hull, Trans.). (2nd ed., Vol. 8) Princeton, NJ: Princeton University Press. (Original work published 1928).

Jung, C. G. (1966). Two essays on analytical psychology. In H. Read, M. Fordham, G. Adler, & W. McGuire (Eds.), *The collected works of C. G. Jung* (R. F. C. Hull, Trans.). (2nd ed., Vol. 7, pp. 127–155). Princeton, NJ: Princeton University Press. (Original work published 1953).

Jung, C. G. (1977). Symbols of transformation. In H. Read, M. Fordham, G. Adler, & W. McGuire (Eds.), *The collected works of C. G. Jung* (R. F. C. Hull, Trans.). (2nd ed., Vol. 5, pp. 394–446). Princeton, NJ: Princeton University Press. (Original work published 1956).

Juslin, P. N., & Laukka, P. (2003). Communications of emotions in vocal expression and music performance: Different channels, same code? *Psychological Bulletin, 129*(5), 770–814. Retrieved from EBSCO*host*.

Kalshed, D. (1996). *The inner world of trauma: Archetypal defense of the personal spirit*. New York, NY: Routledge.

Keil, C., & Feld, S. (1994). *Music grooves*. Chicago: University of Chicago Press.

Kestenbaum, C. J. (1986). Thoughts on the precursors of affective and cognitive disturbance in schizophrenia. In D. B. Feinsilver (Ed.), *Towards a comprehensive model for Schizophrenic Disorders. Psychoanalytic essays in memory of Ping-Nie-Pao* (pp. 211–236). Hillsdale, NJ: Analytic Press.

Khantzian, E. J. (1995). Self-regulation vulnerabilities in substance abusers: Treatment implications. *The Psychology and Treatment of Addictive Behaviors, 2*, 17–41.

Kierkegaard, S. (1954). *The sickness unto death*. (Lowrie, W. Trans.). New York, NY: Anchor edition.

Kingdon, D. G., & Turkington, D. (2005). *Cognitive psychotherapy of schizophrenia*. New York, NY: Guilford.

Klein. M. (1948). A contribution to the theory of anxiety and guilt. *International Journal of Psycho-Analysis, 29*, 114–123. Retrieved from EBSCO*host*.

Klein. M. (1986c). Notes on some schizoid mechanisms. In J. Mitchell (Ed.). *The selected Melanie Klein* (pp. 175–200). New York, NY: The Free Press (Original work published 1946).

Knafo, D. (2012). *Dancing with the unconscious: The art of psychoanalysis and the psychoanalysis of art*. New York: Routledge.

Knoblauch, S. H. (2000). *The musical edge of therapeutic dialogue*. Hillsdale, NJ: The Analytic Press.

Knoblauch, S. H. (2005). Body rhythms and the unconscious: Toward an expanding of clinical attention. *Psychoanalytic Dialogues, 15*(6), 807–827. Retrieved from EBSCO*host*.

Koehler, B. (2003). Interview with Gaetano Benedetti, MD. *Journal of the American Academy of Psychoanalysis, 31*(1), 75–87. Retrieved from PEP Archive database.

Koenig, H. (2009). Research on religion, spirituality, and mental health: A Review. *Canadian Journal of Psychiatry, 54*(5), 283–291. Retrieved from Academic Search Premier database.

Kohut, H. (1957). Observations of the psychological functions of music. *Journal of the American Psychoanalytic Association*, 5389–5407. Retrieved from EBSCO*host*.

Kohut, H. (1972). Thoughts on narcissism and narcissistic rage. In P. Ornstein (Ed.), *The search for the self, 3* (pp. 615–658). Madison, CT: International Universities Press.

Kohut, H. and Levarie S. (1950). On the enjoyment of listening to music. *Psychoanalytic Quarterly, 19*: 64–87.

Konecni, V. (2008). Does music induce emotion? A theoretical and methodological analysis. *Psychology of Aesthetics, 2*(2), 115–129. doi:10.1037/1931-3896.2.2.115.

Kossoff, J. (2009, July 20). Apollo 11 moon landing: Moon music. *The Telegraph*. Retrieved from http://www.telegraph.co.uk.

Kramer, J. (2004). Foreword: a musician listens to a psychoanalyst listening to music. In G. J. Rose, *Between couch and piano: Psychoanalysis, music, art and neuroscience*. New York, NY: Brunner-Routledge.

Krishnan, A., & Berry, J. W. (1992). Acculturative stress and acculturation attitudes among Indian immigrants to the United States. *Psychology and Developing Societies*, *4*(2), 187–212. doi:10.1177/097133369200400206.

Lachman, F. M. (2001). Chapter 14 words and music. *Progress in Self-Psychology*, *17*, 167–178. Retrieved from PepWeb.

Lackey, J., Lovett, R., Wallace, Z. & Logan, M. (2007). Get it Shawty [Performed by Lloyd]. On *Street Love*. [Digital download]. Santa Monica, CA: Universal.

Lacourse, E., Claes, M., & Villeneuve, M. (2001). Heavy metal music and adolescent suicide. *Journal of Youth and Adolescence*, *30*(3), 321. Retrieved from EBSCO*host*.

Langer, S. K. (2009). *Philosophy in a new key: A study in the symbolism of reason, rite, and art*. Boston, MA: Harvard University Press (1942).

Langer, S. K. (1953). *Feeling and form*. New York: Charles Scribner's and Sons.

Langs, R. (1983). *Unconscious communication in everyday life*. New York, NY: Jason Aronson.

Le Clezlio, J. M. G. (1971). *Hai*. Geneva, Switz: Skira.

Leff, J., & Vaughn, C. (1985). *Expressed emotion in families*. New York, NY: Guilford Press.

Leite T. (2003). Music psychotherapy in groups with acute psychotic patients. *International Journal of Psychotherapy*, *8*(2), 117–128. Retrieved from EBSCO*host*.

Lennon, J. (1971). Imagine. On *Imagine* [CD]. New York: NY. Apple.

Lerdahl, F., & Jackendoff, R. (1983). *A generative theory of tonal music*. Cambridge, MA: MIT Press.

Lewis, L. (2004). Mourning, insight, and reduction of suicide risk in schizophrenia. *Bulletin of the Menninger Clinic*, *68*(3), 231–244. Retrieved from EBSCO*host*.

Liebkind, K. (1996) Acculturation and stress. Vietnamese refugees in Finland. *Journal of Cross Cultural Psychology*, *27*, 161–180. Retrieved from EBSCO*host*.

Lopez, J, Winans, M., Combs, J., Jones, M. L., Knight, J., Anderson, K., Shropshire, A., & Jamison, M. (2002). Walking on sunshine [Recorded by J. Lopez]. On *Walking on sunshine* [Digital download]. NY, NY: Epic.

Luhrmann, T. M. (2007). Social defeat and the culture of chronicity: or, why schizophrenia does so well over there and so badly here. *Culture, Medicine & Psychiatry*, *31*(2), 135–172. doi:10.1007/s11013-007-9049-z.

Macpherson, C. (1994). Changing patterns of commitment to island homelands. A case study of Western Samoa. *Pacific Studies*, *17*, 83–116.

Mageo, J. (2008). Zones of ambiguity and identity politics in Samoa. *Journal of the Royal Anthropological Institute*, *14*(1), 61–78. doi:10.1111/j.1467-9655.2007.00478.x.

Malloch, S. N. (2000). Mothers and infants and communicative musicality. *Musicae Scientiae*, *3*(1 suppl.), 29–57.

Malloch, S., & Trevarthen, C. (Eds.) (2009). *Communicative musicality: Exploring the basis of human companionship*. Oxford, UK: Oxford University Press.

Marley, B. & Mayfield, C. (1984). One love [Performed by Bob Marley & The Wailers]. On *Legend* [Digital download]. Kingston, Jamaica: United Island Records.

Martin, G., Clarke, M., & Pearce, C. (1993). Adolescent suicide: Music preference as an indicator of vulnerability. *Journal of the American Academy of Child & Adolescent Psychiatry, 32*(3), 530–535. doi:10.1097/00004583-199305000-00007.

Martindale, C., & Moore, K. (1989). Relationship of musical preference to collative, ecological, and psychophysical variables. *Music Perception, 6*(4), 431–445. Retrieved from EBSCO*host*.

McDade, T. W., & Worthman, C. M. (2004). Socialization ambiguity in Samoan adolescents: A model for human development and stress in the context of culture Change. *Journal of Research on Adolescence (Blackwell Publishing Limited), 14*(1), 49–72. doi:10.1111/j.1532-7795.2004.01401003.x.

McDonald, M. (1970). Transitional tunes and musical development. *Psychoanalytic Study of the Child,* 25: 503–520.

McDougall, J. (1978). Primitive communication and the use of countertransference—reflections on early psychic trauma and its transference effects. *Contemporary Psychoanalysis, 14,* 173–209. Retrieved from EBSCO*host*.

McDougall, J. (1986). *Theatres of the mind: Illusion and truth on the psychoanalytic stage.* London, UK: Free Association Books.

McDougall, J. (1989). *Theaters of the body: A psychoanalytic approach to psychosomatic illness.* New York: W.W. Norton & Co.

McEwen, B. S. (2003). Early life influences on life-long patterns of behavior and health. *Mental Retardation & Developmental Disabilities Research Reviews, 9*(3), 149–154. doi:10.1002/mrdd.10074.

McGorry, P. D., Chanen, A., McCarthy, E., & Van Riel, R. (1991). Posttraumatic stress disorder following recent-onset psychosis: An unrecognized postpsychotic syndrome. *Journal of Nervous and Mental Disease, 179*(5), 253–258. doi:10.1097/00005053-199105000-0000.

McGorry, P., Killackey, E., Elkins, K., Lambert, M., & Lambert, T. (2003). Summary Australian and New Zealand clinical practice guideline for the treatment of schizophrenia (2003). *Australasian Psychiatry, 11*(2), 136–147. doi:10.1046/j.1039-8562.2003.00535.x.

McGorry, P. D., & Yung, A. R. (2003). Early intervention in psychosis: an overdue reform. *Australian & New Zealand Journal of Psychiatry, 37*(4), 393–398. doi:10.1046/j.1440-1614.2003.01192.x.

Mendelssohn, F. (1834). Song Without Words No. 1 in E Major [Recorded by G. Gould]. On *Glenn Gould and* serenity [CD]. New York: Sony Classical. (2003)

Mendelssohn, F. (1830). Song without words no. 9 in E major [Recorded by G. Gould]. On *Glenn Gould and serenity* [CD]. New York, NY: Sony Classical. (2003)

Mickel, E., & Mickel, C. (2002). Family therapy in transition: Choice theory and music. *International Journal of Reality Therapy, 21*(2), 37–40. Retrieved from EBSCO*host*.

Miluk-Kolasa, B., Matejek, M., & Stupnicki, R. (1996). The effects of music listening on changes in selected physiological parameters in adult pre-surgical patients. *Journal of Music Therapy, 33*(3), 208–218. Retrieved from EBSCO*host*.

Mindell, A. (1988). *City shadows.* London, UK: Arkana.

Molino, J. (2000). Toward an evolutionary theory of music and language. In N. L. Wallin, B. Merker, S. Brown, N. L. Wallin, B. Merker, & S. Brown (Eds.), *The origins of music* (pp. 165–176). Cambridge, MA: MIT Press. Retrieved from EBSCO*host*.

Montgomery, G. T. (1992). Acculturation, stressors, and somatization patterns among students from extreme south Texas. *Hispanic Journal of Behavioral Sciences*, *14*(4), 434–454. doi:10.1177/073998639201440.

Moore, T., Zammit, S., Lignford-Hughes, A., Barnes, T., Jones, P. B., Burke, M., & Lewis, G. (2007). Cannabis use and risk of psychotic or affective mental health outcomes: a systematic review. *Lancet*, *370*(9584), 319–328. Retrieved from EBSCO*host*.

Morrison, A. P., Frame, L., & Larkin, W. (2003). Relationships between trauma and psychosis: A review and integration. *British Journal of Clinical Psychology*, *42*(4), 331–353. Retrieved from EBSCO*host*.

Mössler, K., Chen, X., Heldal, T. O., & Gold, C. (2011). Music therapy for people with schizophrenia and schizophrenia-like disorders. *The Cochrane Library*.

Mulvihill, D. (2005). The health impact of childhood trauma: An interdisciplinary review, 1997–2003. *Issues in Comprehensive Pediatric Nursing*, *28*(2), 115–136. doi:10.1080/01460860590950890.

Nagel, J. J. (2007). Melodies of the Mind: Mozart in 1778. *American Imago* (Aural Road Edition), *64*(1), 23–36.

Nagel, J. J. (2008a). Psychoanalytic Perspectives on music: An Intersection on the oral and aural road. *The Psychoanalytic Quarterly*, *77*(2), 507–30.

Nagel, J. J. (2008b). Psychoanalytic and musical perspectives on shame in Donizetti's Lucia di Lammermoor. *Journal of the American Psychoanalytic Association*, *56*(2), 551–63.

Nagel, J. J. (2010, August). Melodies in my mind. The Polyphoney of mental life. *Journal of the American Psychoanalytic Association*, *58*(4), 648–62. (Gertrude and Ernst Ticho Memorial Lecture presented in Washington, D. D., June 11, 2010.

Nagel, J. J. (2013). *Melodies of the mind: connections between psychoanalysis and music*. New York: Routledge.

Narter, M. (2006). The change in the daily knowledge of madness in Turkey. *Journal for the Theory of Social Behaviour*, *36*(4), 409–424. doi:10.1111/j.1468-5914.2006.00314.x.

National Collaborating Centre for Mental Health. (2010). *The NICE guideline on core interventions in the treatment and management of schizophrenia in adults in primary and secondary care* (Updated ed.). Leicester: The British Psychological Society and The Royal College of Psychiatrists. Retrieved from http://www.nccmh.org.uk/.

Neilzen, S. & Cesarec, Z. (1981). On the perception of emotional meaning in music. *Psychology of Music*, *9*, 7–31.

Nijenhuis, E. S. (2004). *Somatoform dissociation: Phenomena, measurement, & theoretical issues*. New York, NY: W. W. Norton. Retrieved from EBSCO*host*.

Noy, P. (1967). The psychodynamics of music. *Journal of Music Theapy*, *4*(2), 45–51.

Noy, P. (1993). How music conveys emotion. In S. Feder, R. Karmel, & G. Pollock (Eds.), *Psychoanalytic explorations of music* (pp. 125–149). Madison, CT: International Universities Press.

Olivier, K. (2006). *Usefulness of embodiment in psychotherapy: Dramatherapy applies neuroscience's knowledge about somatic memoreis.* Concordia University, Department of Creative Arts Therapies, Montreal.

O'Meara, J. T. (1990). *Samoan planters: Tradition and economic development in Polynesia.* Fort Worth, TX: Holt, Rinehart & Winston.

Ostwald, P. (1997). *The ecstasy and tragedy of genius: Glenn Gould.* New York, NY: W. W. Norton.

Owens, P. L., Mutter, R., & Stocks, C. (2010) Mental health and substance abuse-related emergency eepartment visits among adults, 2007. *Statistical Brief #92, Agency for Healthcare Research and Quality.* http://www.hcupus.ahrq.gov/reports/statbriefs/sb92.jsp Retrieved from web 08.06.12.

Ozdas, A., Shiavi, R. G., Wilkes, D. M., Silverman, M. K., & Silverman, S. E. (2004). Analysis of vocal tract characteristics for near-term suicidal risk assessment. *Methods Inf Med, 43*(1), 36–38.

Ozturk, O. M., & Volkan, V. D. (1971). The theory and practice of psychiatry in Turkey. *American Journal of Psychotherapy, 25*(2), 240–271. Retrieved from EBSCO*host.*

Page, J., & Plant, R. (1971). Going to California. On *Led Zeppelin IV* [Digital download]. Headley Grange, UK: Atlantic.

Palmer, R. (1987, September 13). Mick Jagger returns, domesticated. *The New York Times.* Retrieved from http://www.nytimes.com.

Panksepp, J. (2008). The power of the word may reside in the power of affect. *Integrative Psychological and Behavioral Science, 42*(1), 47–55.

Panksepp, J., & Trevarthen, C. (2009). The neuroscience of emotion in music. In S. Malloch & S. Trevarthen (Eds.), *Communicative musicality: Exploring the basis of human companionship,* 105–146. New York: Oxford University Press.

Pareles, J. (2001, October 6). Pop review: Flailing wildly to escape the darkness. *The New York Times,* p. 21. Retrieved from EBSCO*host.*

Patel, A. D. (2008). *Music, language and the brain.* New York: Oxford University Press.

Peccecia, M., & Benedetti, G. (1998). The integration of sensorial channels through progressive mirror drawing in the psychotherapy of schizophrenic patients with disturbances in verbal language. *Journal of the American Academy of Psychoanalysis, 26*(1), 109–122. Retrieved from EBSCO*host.*

Plato. (1977). *Timaeus and Critias.* (D. Lee, Trans.). London, UK: Penguin.

Porcaro, S., & Bettis, J. (1982). Human Nature [Recorded by M. Jackson]. On *Thriller* [Digital download]. Los Angeles, CA: EPIC (1983).

Prezekop, P., & Lee, T. (2009). Persistent psychosis associated with salvia divinorum use. *American Journal of Psychiatry, 166*(7), 832. doi:10.1176/appi.ajp.2009.08121759.

Prine, J. (2000). Angel from Montgomery. On *Souvenirs* [Digital download]. Los Angeles, CA: Oh Boy Records.

Ravel, M. (1899). Pavane pour une infante defuntè [Recorded by K. Jean & Slavic Radio Symphony Orchestra]. On *Chill with Ravel* [CD]. Paris, FR: Naxos. (2004).
Read, J., Mosher, L., & Bentall, R. P. (2004). *Models of madness: Psychological, social biological approaches to schizophrenia.* London, UK: Brunner-Rutledge.
Reading, B., & Birchwood, M. (2005). Early intervention in psychosis: Rationale and evidence for effectiveness. *Disease Management & Health Outcomes, 13*(1), 53–63. Retrieved from EBSCO*host.*
Ready, T. (2010). Music as language, *American Journal of Hospice and Palliative Medicine, 27*(1), 7–15.
Ready, T. (2011). Containment and communication through musical preference, *Music and Medicine, 10*(3), 246–257.
Ready, T. (2013) The listening room, In J. Mondanaro & G. Sara (Eds.), *Music and medicine: Integrative models in pain medicine.* New York, NY: Satchmo Press.
Ready, T. (2014). Sounding home. In M. O'Loughlin & M. Charles (Eds.), *Fragments of trauma and the social production of suffering.* Lanham, MD: Rowman & Littlefield Publishers.
Redding, O., & Cropper, S. (1968). Dock of the Bay [Recorded by O. Redding]. On *Dock of the Bay* [Digital Download]. Memphis, TN: Volt/ATCO.
Reich, W. (1972). *Character analysis* (3rd ed., V. R. Garfagno. Trans.). New York, NY: Farrar, Strauss & Giroux. (Original work published 1945).
Reich, W. (1973). *Selected writings: An introduction to orgonomy.* New York, NY: Farrar, Strauss & Giroux. (Original work published 1951).
Reik, T. (1953). *The haunting melody: Psychoanalytic experiences in life and music.* New York: Farrar, Strauss and Young.
Rideout, V., Foehr, U. G., & Roberts, D. F. (2010, January). Gen M2: Media in the lives of 8 to 18 year olds. *A Kaiser Family Foundation Study.* Retrieved from Kaiser Family Foundation 2014 http:cmch.tv/parents/music.
Robinson, D. G., Woerner, M. G., Alvir, J. M. J., et al. (1999). Predictors of treatment response from a first episode of schizophrenia or schizoaffective disorder. *American Journal of Psychiatry, 156*(4), 544–549. Retrieved from EBSCO*host.*
Robinson, M. (2010). *Absence of mind.* New Haven, CT: Yale Press.
Rose, G. (1996). *Necessary illusion: Art as witness.* Madison, CT: International Universities Press.
Rose, G. (2004). *Between couch and piano.* New York: Brunner-Routledge.
Rosenbaum, B. (2005). Psychosis and the structure of homosexuality: Understanding the pathogenesis of schizophrenic states of mind. *Scandinavian Psychoanalytic Review, 28*(2), 82–89. Retrieved from EBSCO*host.*
Rosenbaum, B., & Harder, S. (2007). Psychosis and the dynamics of the psychotherapy process. *International Review of Psychiatry, 19*(1), 13–23.
Rosenblum, D. S., Daniolos, P, Kass, N. & Martin, A. (1999). Adolescents and Popular Culture. *Psychoanalytic Study of Children, 54*: 319–338.
Rubin, S. S., & Niemeier, D. L. (1992). Non-verbal affective communication as a factor in psychotherapy. *Psychotherapy: Theory, Research, Practice, Training, 29*(4), 596–602. doi:10.1037/0033-3204.29.4.596.

Rubinstein, D. H. (1983). Epidemic suicide among Micronesian adolescents. *Social Science & Medicine, 17*(10), 657–665. doi:10.1016/0277-9536(83)90372-6.

Ruby, P., & Decety, J. (2001). Effect of subjective perspective taking during simulation of action: A PET investigation of agency. *Nature Neuroscience, 4*(5), 546–550. Retrieved from EBSCO*host*.

Sachs, L. (1983). Evil eye or bacteria: Turkish migrant women and Swedish health care. *Stockholm: Studies in Social Anthopology*, 64–65.

Sacks, O. (2007). *Musicophilia: Tales of music and the brain*. New York, NY: Alfred A. Knopf.

Sam, D. L., & Berry, J. W. (1995). Acculturative stress among young immigrants in Norway. *Scandinavian Journal of Psychology, 36*(1), 10–24. doi:10.1111/j.1467-9450.1995.tb00964.

Samuels, A. (1985). Countertransference, The "Mundus Imaginalis" and a research project. *Journal of Analytical Psychology, 30*(1), 47–71. Retrieved from EBSCO*host*.

Santayana, G. (1955). *The sense of beauty: Being the outline of aesthetic theory*. New York, NY: Dover Publications, Inc.

Schoeffel, P. (2000). Theorising self in Samoa, emotions, genders and sexualities (Book Review). *Oceania, 71*(2), 161. Retrieved from Academic Search Premier database.

Schore, A. N. (1994). *Affect regulation and the origins of the self*. Mahwah, NJ: Lawrence Erlbaum.

Schore, A. N. (2001). Effects of a secure attachment relationship on right brain development, affect regulation, and infant mental health. *Infant Mental Health Journal, 22*(1/2), 7–66. Retrieved from EBSCO*host*.

Schore, A. N. (2002). Implications of a psychoneurological model. In S. Alhanti (Ed.), *Primitive mental states (Vol 2): Psychobiological and psychoanalytic perspectives on early trauma and personality development* (pp. 1–64), New York, NY: Karnac.

Schulkind, M. D., Hennis, L., & Rubin, D. C. (1999). Music, emotion, and autobiographical memory: They're playing your song. *Memory & Cognition, 27*(6), 948–955. Retrieved from EBSCO*host*.

Schubert, E. (2010). Affective, evaluative, and collative responses to hated and loved music. *Psychology of Aesthetics, Creativity, and the Arts, 4*(1), 36–46. doi:10.1037/a0016316.

Searles, H. F. (1979). *Countertransference and related subjects*. New York, NY: International Universities Press, Inc.

Silverman, M. J. (2003). The influence of music on the symptoms of psychosis: a meta-analysis. *Journal of Music Therapy, 40*(1), 27–40.

Szegedy-Maszak, M. (2004). Emergency of the mind. *U.S. News & World Report, 136*(16), 62.

Seligman, L., & Reichenber, L. W. (2007). *Selecting effective treatments: A comprehensive, systematic guide to treating mental disorders*. San Francisco, CA: Jossey-Bass.

Selten, J., & Cantor-Graae, E. (2004). Schizophrenia and migration. In W. Gattaz, & H. Hafner, *Search for the causes of schizophrenia* (Vol. 5, pp. 3–25). Darnstadt, DE: Springer/Steinkopf Verlag.

Simmon, E., & Storch, S. (2006). Lord give me a sign [Recorded by DMX]. On *Lord give me a sign* [CD]. New York, NY: Ruff Ryders.

Skar, P. (2002). The goal as process: Music and the search for the Self. *Journal of Analytical Psychology, 47*(4), 629–638. Retrieved from EBSCO*host*.

Slade, M. (2009). *Personal recovery and mental illness. A guide for mental health professionals*. Cambridge: Cambridge University Press.

Sluckin, W. W., Hargreaves, D. J., & Colman, A. M. (1982). Some experimental studies of familiarity and liking. *Bulletin of the British Psychological Society, 351*, 89–194. Retrieved from EBSCO*host*.

Sokolova, A. N. (2006). Music as medicine: The Adygh's case. In D. Aldridge & J. Fachner (Eds.), *Music and altered states: Consciousness, transcendence, therapy and addictions* (pp. 74–81). Philadelphia: Jessica Kingsley.

Solli, H. P., & Rolvsjord, R. (2015). The opposite of treatment: A qualitative study of how patients diagnosed with psychosis experience music therapy. *Nordic Journal of Music Therapy, 24*(1), 67–92.

Solomon, A. (2001). *The noonday demon: An atlas of depression*. New York, NY: Simon & Schuster.

Sperber, M. (1999). Variations on a theme of shame: Chekhov, Glenn Gould, and the "Cased-in-man" syndrome. *Psychoanalytic Review, 86*(2), 175–189. Retrieved from EBSCO*host*.

Stack, S. (1998). Heavy metal, religiosity, and suicide acceptability. *Suicide & Life-Threatening Behavior, 28*(4), 388–394. Retrieved from EBSCO*host*.

Stern, D. N. (1985). *The interpersonal world of the infant*. New York: Basic Books.

Stern, D. N. (1995). The motherhood constellation. New York, NY: Basic Books.

Spotnitz, H. (2004), *Modern psychoanalysis of the schizophrenic patient: Theory of the technique* (2nd Ed.). New York, NY: YBK.

Stolorow, D. S., & Stolorow, R. D. (1987). Affects and self objects. In R. D. Stolorow, B. Brandschaft, & E. Atwood (Eds.), *Psychoanalytic treatment: An intersubjective approach* (pp. 66–87). Hillsdale, NJ: Analytic Press.

Stone, J., Child, D., Wright, B. (2004). Right to be wrong. On *Mind Body & Soul*. [Digital download] New York, NY: Relentless.

Stone, M. (2006). The analyst's body as tuning fork: Embodied resonance in countertransference. *Journal of Analytical Psychology, 51*(1), 109–124. Retrieved from EBSCO*host*.

Storr, A. (1992). *Music and the mind*. New York, NY: Ballantine Books.

Strauss, R. (1881). Sonata for piano in B minor, Op. 5 [Recorded by G. Gould]. On *Glenn Gould and serenity* [CD]. New York, NY: Sony Classical. (2003)

Stuart, T. (2015). Personal email from President of the Wagner Society of Northern California.

Sunter, A. T., Guz, H., & Peksen, Y. (2006). The search for non-medical treatment for patients with psychiatric disorders. *Journal of Religion and Health, 3*(Fall), 393–404.

Tarrant, M., North, A. C., & Hargreaves, D. J. (2000). English and American adolescents' reasons for listening to music. *Psychology of Music, 28*(2), 166–173. doi:10.1177/0305735600282005.

Taylor, J. (1971). You can close your eyes [Recorded by Carole King and James Taylor]. On *Live at the Troubador* [Digital download]. West Hollywood, CA: Hear Music.

Tekman, H. G., & Hortacsu, N. (2002). Music and social identity: Stylistic identification as a response to musical style. *International Journal of Psychology, 37*(5), 277–285. doi:10.1080/00207590244000043.

The Norwegian Directorate of Health. (2013). *Nasjonal faglig retningslinje for utredning, behandling og oppfølging av personer med psykoselidelser* [National guidelines for assessment, treatment, and follow-up of persons with psychotic illnesses]. Oslo: Author. Retrieved from http://helsedirektoratet.no/.

Theuma, M., Read, J., Moskowitz, A., & Stewart, A. (2007). Evaluation of a New Zealand early intervention service for psychosis. *New Zealand Journal of Psychology, 36*(3), 136–145. Retrieved from PsycINFO database.

Thiele, B. & Weiss, G. D. (1967). What a wonderful world [Recorded by Israel "IZ" Ka'ano'i Kamakawiwo'ole]. On *Wonderful world* [CD]. Honolulu, HI: Mountain Apple. (2007)

Thornton, A., Kerslake, M., & Binns, T. (2010). Alienation and obligation: Religion and social change in Samoa. *Asia Pacific Viewpoint, 51*(1), 1–16. doi:10.1111/j.1467-8373.2010.01410.x.

Tomkins, S. (1962). Affect, imagery, consciousness, Vol. 1: *The positive affects*, New York: Springer-Verlag.

Tool (2001b). The patient. On *Lateralus* [Digital download]. Hollywood, CA: Volcanoe Entertainment.

Trevarthen, C. (1999). How music heals. In T. Wigram, & J. De-Backer (Eds.), *Clinical applications of music therapy in developmental disability; pediatrics and neurology*. London, UK: Jessica Kingsley.

Trevarthen, C. (2005). First things first: infants make good use of the sympathetic rhythm of imitation, without reason or language. *Journal of Child Psychotherapy, 31*(1), 91–113.

Trevarthen, C., & Aitken, K. J. (1995). Brain development, infant communication and empathy disorders. Intrinsic factors in child mental health. *Development and Psychopathology*, 6: 597–633.

Trevarthen, C., & Malloch, S. N. (2000). The dance of well-being: Defining the musical therapeutic effect. *Nordic Journal of Music Therapy, 9*(1), 13–17. doi:10.1080/08098130009477996.

Tronick, E. Z., & Cohn, J. F. (1989). Infant-mother face-to-face interaction: Age and gender differences in coordination and the occurrence of miscoordination. *Child development*, 85–92.

Tustin, F. (1972). *Autism* and *childhood psychosis*. London: Hogarth.

Twemlow, S. (2009). Cmmentary on Isaac Tylims Paper. *International Journal of Applied Psychoanalytic Studies, 6*(1), 93.

Ulrich, G., Houtmans, T. & Gold, C. (2007). The additional therapeutic effect of group music therapy for schizophrenic patients: a randomized study. *Acta Psychiatrica Scandinavica, 116*(5), 362–370. doi:10.1111/j.1600-0447.2007.01073.x

Usher, da Don, P., Young Jeezy, Taylor, L., Lovett, R., Thomas, K., & Dalton, D. (2008). Love in this club. On *Here I stand* [Digital Download]. Atlanta, GA: La Face.

van der Kolk, B., McFarlane, A., & Weisaeth, L. (Eds.) (1996). *Traumatic stress. The effects of overwhelming experience on mind, body and society.* New York and London: Guilford.

van der Kolk, B., Roth, S., Pelcovitz, D., Sunday, S. & Spinazzola, J. (2005). Disorders of extreme stress: The empirical foundation of a complex adaptation to trauma *Journal of Traumatic Stress, 18*(5), 389–399. Retrieved from EBSCO*host.*

Vega, S. (1986). Marlene on the Wall. On *Suzanne Vega* [Digital download]. New York, NY: UMG Records.

Vega, S. (1987a). Luka. On *Solitude Standing* [Digital download]. New York, NY: A & M.

Vega, S. (1987b). Solitude standing. On *Solitude standing* [Digital download]. New York, NY: A & M.

Vega, S. (1987c). Tom's diner. [Recorded by S. Vega]. On *Solitude standing* [Digital Download]. New York, NY: A & M.

Vega, S. (2003). Calypso. [Recorded by S. Vega]. On *Retrospective: The best of Suzanne Vega* [Digital download]. New York, NY: Interscope Geffen.

Vivaldi, A. (1741). Cum dederit delectis suis somnum. [Recorded by Australian Brandenburg Orchestra, & P. Dyer]. On *Baraoque adagios* [CD]. New York, NY: Universal Classics Group. (2002)

Wiederhorn. (1996). Tool get spiritual and scatological with "aenima." *Rolling Stone, 748*(41), http://www.rollingstone.com.

Williams, S. (2002). Not in our name [Recorded by S. Williams, & D. J. Spooky]. On *Not in our name* [Digital download]. New York, NY: Synchronicity.

Winkler, I., Haden, G., Lading, O., Sziller. I., & Honing, H. (2009). Newborn infants detect the beat in music. Retrieved from *The National Academy of Sciences of the USA*: www.pnas.org/cgi/doi/10.1073/pnas.0809035106.

Winnicott D. W. (1953). Transitional objects and transitional phenomena. *International Journal of Psychoanalysis, 34:* 89–97.

Winnicott, D. W. (1958). *Through paediatrics to pscyho-analysis: Collected papers.* New York: Basic Books.

Winnicott, D. W. (1968). Playing: Its theoretical status in the clinical situation. *International Journal of Psychoanalysis, 49,* 591–599. Retrieved from EBSCO*host.*

Winnicott, D. W. (1971). *Playing and reality.* London, UK: Routledge.

Winnicott, D. W. (1974). Fear of Breakdown. *International Review of Psychoanalysis, 1,* 103–107.

Wittmann, D., & Keshavan, M. (2007). Grief and mourning in schizophrenia. *Psychiatry: Interpersonal & Biological Processes, 70*(2), 154–166. Retrieved from Academic Search Premier database.

Wright, J. H., Turkington, D., Kingdon, D, & Ramirez Basco, M. (2009). *Cognitive-behavior therapy for severe mental illness.* Washington, DC: American Psychiatric Publishing.

Yorke, T., & Greenwood, J. (2007a). Nude [Recorded by Radiohead]. On *In rainbows* [Digital download]. London, UK: _Xurbia_Xendless, Ltd.

Yorke, T., & Greenwood, J. (2007b). Weird Fishes/Arpeggi [Recorded by Radiohead]. On *In rainbows* [Digital download]. London, UK: _Xurbia_Xendless, Ltd.

Index

abandonment, fear of, 19, 21, 30, 54, 64
abuse, impact of, 3, 38, 63–65, 69, 71, 79
adolescents, 11–12, 14, 50.
 See also young adults
affect states, 1, 25;
 contained through music, 12, 30, 63, 76;
 expressed through music, 9–11, 49
alpha function. *See under* Bion, Wilfred
annihilation:
 fantasy of, 33, 44;
 fear of, 13, 26, 30, 33, 66, 67, 86
anxiety, 12, 21, 50, 55, 67, 79;
 music and, 14–15, 19, 45, 53–54, 79, 84–86
Aron, Lewis, 85
art, 9, 72, 79
attachment, 69;
 disrupted, 13;
 mother's body and, 9–10;
 musical elements in, 9, 14, 24;
 music as attachment object, 18, 76
attunement, 3–4, 8, 10, 12, 20, 25, 61;
 music and, 15, 18, 21, 24, 54, 57, 58, 61, 67, 84–85

Bach, Johann Sebastian, 3, 28–29, 31–32, 34, 58, 79, 83, 85
baroque music, effects of, 28, 34, 77, 84

Beebee, Beatrice, 4, 10, 18, 20–21, 78
Beethoven, Ludwig van, 9, 22–23, 32, 67, 83, 85
Benedetti, Gaetano, 49–50, 56, 61, 80
Benjamin, Jessica, 20
Bentall, Richard P., 38, 50
Bion, Wilfred, 2, 4, 11, 13–15, 20, 23, 25–26, 28, 30, 36, 39, 54;
 alpha function, 25, 41, 75;
 attacking links, 61;
 hallucinosis, 26, 77;
 metabolization, 25–26, 72, 74, 83;
 nameless dread, 25;
 psychosis, 41, 65;
 therapeutic dyad, 67, 84
bipolar disorder, 3, 5, 13, 22, 27, 50
Birchwood, Max, 50
body, 2, 8, 10, 59, 66, 84–85;
 autonomic response, 10;
 gesture as communication, 64–65;
 physiological symptoms, 13, 40;
 primitive body states, 39, 66;
 rhythmo–affective semantics, 2;
 threshold capacity, 13, 41;
 unconscious communication and, 39, 66, 85;
 violence toward, 51, 64.
 See also brain, music and
borderline personality disorder, 8, 13, 79–80

brain, music and, 61, 23, 75;
    intersubjective collaboration and, 18;
    right hemisphere, role of, 10, 41
Bucci, Wilma, 2, 13

Campbell, Christine, 19, 51, 75
Carter, Jr., Dwayne Michael.
    See Lil Wayne
Charles, Marilyn, 26, 39, 57
classical music, 2;
    calming effects of, 55, 77;
    negative response to, 23, 79;
    preference for, 35;
    psychoanalytic tradition and, 2, 9;
    psychosis, impact of classical music on, 85;
    tolerance for, 79;
    young adults and, 14
communicative musicality, 10, 20, 74
countertransference, 18, 34, 38–39, 48, 58–59, 61, 66, 70, 85–86;
    embodied countertransference, 38, 66

Darwin, Charles, 3
Davis, Miles, 55, 83
Davoine, Françoise, 39, 43, 72
depression, 45, 50, 58, 66, 76
Derulo, Jason, 70–71
Dileo, Cheryl, 8
Dion, Celine, 19, 21
Dissanayake, Ellen, 8
dissonance, 19, 24, 54–55, 58, 61, 64, 84
drug use:
    alcohol, 57, 61;
    designer drugs, 61;
    marijuana, 49, 51, 60;
    music for counterbalancing, 50;
    recreational, 22, 49;
    salvia divinorum, 60

early psychosis intervention, 22, 49–51
Ehrzenweig, Anton, 9
Eigen, Mike, 35, 65, 86
Ekman, Paul, 10
Emde, Robert N., 10

Eminem, 75
emotional regulation, 3, 10, 12–14, 18, 21, 23, 25–26, 44, 52, 76, 78–79

Feder, Stuart, 10–11
Freud, Sigmund, 3, 9, 41, 68, 70
Fromm, Erich, 13
Fromm-Reichman, Frieda, 18

Gaudillière, Jean-Max, 39, 43, 72
gender, 56
Glenn Gould, 30–34, 56
Glück, Franz, 56
Gotlib, Ian H., 19, 51
Graf, Max, 9
grief:
    bearing of, 1, 14, 28;
    deferred, 76, 78;
    music in mediation of, 29, 32–34, 36, 44–45, 67, 76
Grotstein, James, 4, 19, 26, 39, 70;
    orphans of the real, 13

hallucinosis, 15, 26, 77
Hargreaves, David J., 4, 50, 81
healing, music and, 66–69, 19, 51;
    Adyghs, 8;
    cultural tradition and, 30–32;
    history of, 8;
    social connection and, 69;
    spiritual aspects of, 30–32, 36
heavy metal, 3, 15, 67, 81
Hippocrates, 8
Hooley, Jill M., 19, 51
Hortacsu, Nuran, 4

"Imagine", 1, 12
inner life, 20, 30;
    music as portal to, 2, 9, 11, 19, 34;
    psychosis and, 39
iPod. *See* portable music device

Jackson, Michael, 22–23, 41–43, 47, 70–71, 77
jazz, 9, 55, 73, 85

Journey, 7, 79
Jung, Carl, 3, 22, 36, 68

Kamakawiwo'ole, Israel, 7, 23, 46
Kierkegaard, Søren, 65
Kingdon, David G., 13, 37–38
Klein, Melanie, 26, 31, 70
Knoblauch, Steven H., 11, 13, 20, 55, 59;
   musical edge, 11, 24;
   process contours, 11
Koehler, Brian, 56, 61, 80
Kohut, Heinz, 9–10, 44, 74
Konečni, Vladimir J., 2, 77
Kramer, Jonathan, 8

Lachman, Frank M., 9–11, 20
Langer, Susan, 11, 20
Lennon, John, 1
Lil Wayne, 43–44, 67, 70–71
listening to music with patients:
   benefits of, 3, 11, 20–21, 23–24, 38, 49, 86;
   building rapport in, 11, 14, 17, 20, 42, 53, 55, 61, 83–86;
   containment and, 14, 25, 35, 52, 67;
   cultural issues and, 71, 86;
   emotional processing and, 4, 14, 25, 29, 32, 56, 71–72, 76;
   equality in, 14, 83–85;
   linking, patient's resistance to, 21, 23, 78;
   metabolization. *See under* Bion;
   mismatch, rematch, and repair, 20, 22, 58;
   openness to patient's music, 11, 20, 84–85, 86;
   organization of patient's self and, 13, 23;
   potential space and, 38, 43, 75;
   safety in, 11, 20, 45, 57, 72, 74, 76;
   social connection, 4, 7, 15, 17, 74, 78;
   translations, 29, 86.
   See also young adults: listening to music with

Loewy, Joanne, 8
lullabies, 9–10, 12, 46

Marley, Bob, 19, 43
Mathers, Marshall. *See* Eminem
McDonald, Marjorie, 12
McDougall, Joyce, 38–39, 43, 48, 66
McEwen, Bruce S., 13, 41
McGorry, Patrick, 4, 22, 49–50
medications, 21–22, 27, 36, 57–58, 60, 68
melody, 5, 10, 53, 67, 81, 86
memory, music and, 3, 13, 62;
   drug use, association with, 23, 61;
   painful memories, 13, 27, 30, 78
Mendelssohn, Franz, 30, 33, 78
Metallica, 3, 67
metaphor as communication, 3, 33, 59, 62, 64, 74
mind:
   emergent sense of self, 18, 22, 48;
   processing, 11, 34, 54–55;
   similarities to music, 11
Molino, Jean, 2
Morrison, Van, 83
mother, 1, 3, 4, 10, 20, 74, 78;
   absence of, 31, 55, 73;
   affect regulation, and, 12, 52;
   attunement with, 3, 4, 9, 10;
   breakdown of raw material, 4, 25, 72;
   lullaby, 9–10, 12, 46;
   metabolization of new experience, 25, 30;
   mother-infant dyad, 4, 5;
   non-verbal communication and, 2, 10, 13;
   similarities to therapist patient dyad, 1, 10 18, 74;
   transference mother, 61;
   voice of, 1, 3, 10, 17, 19, 58.
   See also Bion: alpha function; communicative musicality
Mulvihill, Deanna, 13, 41
music, 3, 9, 14, 33, 51–52, 74–75, 79–80;

addictive features of, 18, 23, 61;
affect expression through, 52, 55, 58, 67, 69, 84;
affect regulation, role in, 3, 12–13, 18, 44, 54;
attunement through, 3, 52, 61, 67, 84–85;
auxiliary mothering function and, 1, 52;
calming effects of, 3, 5, 7–8, 38–39, 52, 74, 77, 79;
communication through, 15, 20, 23, 30, 40, 59–60, 80, 81, 84;
conflicts, mediated by, 12, 14, 34, 36, 52, 55, 57, 59, 69, 71;
containment of emotions and, 9, 21, 36, 40, 55, 61, 67;
creativity and, 59, 72;
cultural aspects of, 26, 27, 31, 35 69, 71, 86;
displacement through, 12, 14, 75;
dream structure, similarity to, 9, 22;
drug-related associations, 24, 55, 61;
emotional awareness and, 11, 21, 23, 52, 59–60;
familiarity of, 10, 74, 81;
fragments of self, in, 19, 28, 34, 75;
framing with, 7, 11–12, 22, 26, 49, 53, 67, 76;
grief, working through with, 1, 28–29, 32–33, 76;
identity and, 11, 12, 49–50, 53, 59–60, 67, 70, 78, 81, 84;
implicit material and, 3, 21, 23, 41, 43, 78, 86–87;
increasing tolerance through, 32, 54, 76–77, 80;
inner life and, 9, 11, 19, 20, 30, 34, 39, 56;
metaphors inspired by, 9, 42, 59;
modulating pain and arousal, 10, 18, 52, 54, 80;
non-verbal expression through, 66, 77–79;
organizing effect of, 12–14, 30, 45, 75, 77, 86;

performance of, 5, 7, 40, 48, 68, 69, 72;
play, music as form of, 12, 42, 54;
potential space and, 8, 37–48, 75, 85;
safety and, 3, 11, 14, 20, 36, 39, 76, 78–79, 84;
self-expression through, 44, 70;
silence, and, 52, 57;
spiritual aspects of, 22, 30–33;
synchronization, 8, 11, 77;
therapist's voice as. *See* voice;
transformation of raw emotions through, 25, 41, 56, 8;
transitional object, 1, 4, 12, 57;
trauma, and, 8, 35, 63, 67–68, 79;
unconscious response to, 1, 3, 9, 14–15, 18, 36, 38, 41, 52, 53, 56, 71, 77–78, 84;
voice-hearing and, 17, 32, 52, 80;
volume, modulation of, 5, 10, 53, 67, 81, 86
musical preference. *See* self-selected music
music groups, 74, 76–78, 80–81
musicians:
as metabolizers of affect, 43–44, 67, 70–71, 74, 75, 77;
as transference objects, 22, 58–59, 71
music therapy, 8

Nagel, Julie Jaffee, 9–11, 15, 18;
on Freud, 9;
oral and aural road, 9–10, 18
Nijenhuis, Ellert R. S., 13
North, Adrian C., 4, 50, 81
Noy, Pinchas, 9, 12

object relations, 31
opera, 2, 9, 62, 85, 87
otherness, 39, 51, 68, 71, 86

Panksepp, Jaak, 4, 18
parataxis, 46
Parker, Courtney, 8
Patel, Aniruddh D., 3, 10
personal listening device, 37, 50, 86;

creation of safe space with, 37,
  79–80;
groups organized around, 7, 77;
individuals with, 49–50, 79–80;
mediation of emotional experience
  with, 79–80;
memorializing experience with, 50,
  57, 80;
symbol for self, 4, 49–50, 86;
transitional object, 86;
as witness, 26
Plato, 8
polyphony in music, 12, 29, 42, 87
popular music, 14, 25, 58;
  body awareness and, 14, 59;
  importance of, 2, 11, 12;
  psychosis reduced with, 85;
  traits associated with, 81.
  See also names of musicians
Portishead, 52, 57
post traumatic stress disorder. *See* PTSD
preferred music.
  See self-selected music
Prine, John, 29
psychiatric hospitalization:
  involuntary, 22, 36, 51, 68;
  as temporary community, 15;
  traumatization in, 27, 38, 61, 68
psychosis, 13, 27, 39, 51, 57, 60, 65;
  attacking linking and, 26, 51, 73,
    77–78;
  boundaries and, 54, 56;
  catharsis through music, 49, 57,
    58, 74;
  cultural aspects of, 27, 31, 35,
    70–71;
  disorganization and, 26, 29, 70;
  disturbances in verbal language, 49,
    70;
  drug use and, 22, 49, 51, 60;
  early psychosis intervention, 4, 49;
  fragmentation in, 30, 70;
  music as form of communication in,
    26–37;
  origins of, 13, 36;
  primary process thinking in, 29, 41;

re-enactment of primal scene and,
  64, 72;
sensitivity to sensory stimulus, 13;
social support, lack of, 2, 41, 70;
splitting, 26, 70;
transcendent urge in, 28, 30;
transformation through regression,
  35, 36;
trauma and, 13, 38, 41, 63;
voice-hearing and, 15, 17, 22, 27, 32,
  38, 53–54, 57, 75, 80
PTSD, 3, 13, 35, 38, 79

Qur'an, 29–32, 34–35

Ravel, Maurice, 28–29
raves, 19, 21, 23, 59, 60
Redding, Otis, 7
Reich, Wilhelm, 39
Reik, Theodore, 9, 11
rhythm, 2, 8, 10, 11–12, 14, 21, 24,
  42–43, 52–53, 55–58, 61, 66,
  77–78, 80–81
Rorschach, 24, 28–29, 35
Rose, Gilbert, 8–9, 13–14, 26, 40
Rosenbaum, Bent, 10, 54

Sacks, Oliver, 8
Schizophrenia, 13, 20, 49, 54, 56,
  60, 75;
  drug use and, 60;
  music's impact on symptoms, 14;
  origins, 13
Schore, Allan, 41
self-selected music, 18, 23, 74;
  agency in choice of, 59;
  borrowing language from, 49;
  communication through, 19, 49, 53;
  containment and, 49, 53, 59;
  diagnoses and, 81;
  emotional expression and, 49;
  emotional regulation using, 19,
    47, 49;
  preferred qualities of music, 81;
  unconscious links and, 52–53
sexual identity, 69

Sinatra, Frank, 28, 32
social bonding with music, 74
social defeat, 70
Solomon, Andrew, 66
Stern, Daniel N., 4, 10, 18, 52, 83
stigma, 23, 59, 86
Stone, Joss, 5
Storr, Anthony, 8
substance use. *See* drug use
suicide, 64–66, 69;
　as exorcism, 66, 71;
　potential of music in crisis, 68;
　pre-suicidal voice pattern, 66;
　re-enactment of abuse and, 64–66, 72;
　social issues and, 67, 69
Sullivan, Harry Stack, 21, 46

Tekman, Hasan Gürkan, 4
therapeutic alliance, 4, 10, 28, 32, 39, 57, 60, 66;
　attunement and, 10, 51, 57–58, 61, 84;
　building immediate rapport, 8;
　call and response in, 12, 20, 53;
　dangers for patient inherent in, 51, 73;
　difficult-to-reach patients, 30, 73, 86;
　equality in, 14, 53, 83, 85;
　frame, 76, 85;
　improvisation in, 83–84;
　linking language in, 26–36;
　metaphor and, 20, 27, 33;
　potential space, tending of, 12, 37, 45, 58;
　shifting base between therapist and patient, 20, 35, 53, 58;
　symbolic communication, 45, 60;
　synchronization, 11, 58;
　syncopation in, 11, 42, 60;
　therapist's metabolization process, 67, 68, 83–84;
　trust-building and, 10, 14, 26, 36, 41, 43, 46, 55, 73, 84;
　unconscious and, 38, 52, 7;

voice and, 11, 51, 53, 58.
　See also transference, countertransference
tone, 11, 13, 18–20, 23, 28, 51–52, 55, 59, 66, 68, 80–81, 84
Tool, 22, 61;
　collective unconscious, 22
transference, 22, 39, 42–44, 52, 55, 58
transitional object, 1, 4, 12
transitional tunes, 12
trauma:
　impact on therapeutic alliance, 13;
　performance of as catharsis, 77–78;
　re-enactment of, 18, 64–65, 72;
　transmission of, 43
Treverathen, Colwyn, 4, 10
Tronick, Edward Z., 20
Turkington, Douglas, 13, 37–38
Tustin, Frances, 39

unconscious, 1, 3, 11, 15, 36, 41, 65, 68;
　associations and, 1, 36, 53;
　attunement to, 38–39, 77, 84;
　communications and, 3, 39;
　conflicts, 14, 71;
　music as portal to, 9, 18, 43–44, 52, 78, 85

van der Kolk, Bessel, 13, 41
Vega, Suzanne, 19, 52
voice, 17, 19, 21, 55, 58–59, 66, 70–72, 75;
　associations and, 1, 10, 17, 43, 58;
　authenticity of, 23, 63, 80–81;
　effect of, 1, 3, 10, 19–21, 22, 34, 64, 86;
　high expressed emotion and, 19, 51;
　musical attunement with, 35, 46, 52, 57, 66;
　therapist's, 11, 51, 58–59, 68

Wagner Richard, 2, 62, 85, 87
Winnicott, Donald, 4, 7, 12, 20–21, 37, 45, 52, 64–65, 72

young adults, 14, 58;
    drug use and, 49;
    globalization and, 35, 70;
    identity formation of, 11;
    indirect communication and, 14;
    listening to music with, 11, 49, 80, 84;
    musical preference and, 81;
    social media, 50, 63, 86
Yo-Yo Ma, 3, 58, 79
Yung Alison R., 4, 22, 50

About the Author

Trisha Ready is a psychologist who manages a partial hospitalization program in Seattle. She received an Honorable Mention in the Johanna K. Tabin book competition for an earlier version of this manuscript. She has had articles published in the *Division/Review, American Journal of Hospice and Palliative Medicine, Music and Medicine,* and *Psychoanalysis, Culture, and Society,* as well as book chapters in *Music and Medicine: Integrative Models in Pain Medicine* and *Fragments of Trauma and the Social Production of Suffering*. Trisha has published other music-based essays in a variety of media. Her essay, "How listening to music and fighting with Susan Sontag helped me cope with chemo," was chosen by *Longreads.com* as one of the best essays of 2015.

Lightning Source UK Ltd.
Milton Keynes UK
UKOW03n0357240217
295214UK00010B/114/P